SUPPORTING QUEER BIRTH

Supporting Queer Birth

A Book for Birth Professionals
and Parents

AJ Silver

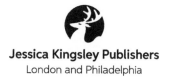

Jessica Kingsley Publishers

London and Philadelphia

First published in Great Britain in 2022 by Jessica Kingsley Publishers
An imprint of Hodder & Stoughton Ltd
An Hachette Company

1

A CIP catalogue record for this title is available from the British Library and the
Library of Congress

ISBN 978 1 83997 045 0
eISBN 978 1 83997 046 7

Printed and bound by CPI Group (UK) Ltd, Croydon, CR0 4YY

Jessica Kingsley Publishers' policy is to use papers that are natural, renewable
and recyclable products and made from wood grown in sustainable forests.
The logging and manufacturing processes are expected to conform to the
environmental regulations of the country of origin.

Jessica Kingsley Publishers
Carmelite House
50 Victoria Embankment
London EC4Y 0DZ

www.jkp.com

Contents

Acknowledgements

My children, Izzy and Emma. Many times, you were told that Bubba was writing, don't go in there! But you came in anyway to tell me about the butterfly, rock or whatever you had seen that just couldn't wait. Thank you.

Dad, Bob Broadbent. 1952–2020

Grapsie, Kay Broadbent. 1928–2021

Mars Lord, for her continual, unwavering support for me and for her commitment to the non-binary and trans community. Too many texts of 'write bitch' were sent and received, followed usually by 'You are dehydrated'. Thank you. I didn't drink enough water.

Abbie, Adam, Adelaide, Ash, Caprice, Freddy, Gina, Helen, Jake, JB, Jen, Kayden, Kevin, Laura-Rose, Mari, Martha, Nathan, Nicki, Rivers, Sabia, Steph and Princess Leia.

Preface

It is so easy to forget why we are even here. Why do we need a book about births outside the cis heteronormative? While cries for all lives matter try to invalidate those of black lives matter, and confused voices search for international men's day, usually only around the time of international women's day, similar voices are raised asking when is Straight Pride. Why do we need an LGBT+ Pride month; why do we need a parade?

The reason? In the developed world, today, we are being killed, we are dying by suicide. We are being fired, we are being evicted, we are being attacked, physically, emotionally and financially, because of who we are, who we love.[1]

In 2020, trans women of colour were the most murdered in our community.[2] We have lesbians beaten and bloodied on London buses because they refused to kiss for men's enjoyment. We have huge restaurant chains in the USA giving millions to charities that discriminate against homosexuality. We have midwifery groups picking venues that prohibit LGBT+ people from attending, let alone speaking. We have protests at school gates when we dare to think that children should learn that we exist, you know, just like they learn that straight people exist. Across the world, from Ukraine to Tanzania, from Russia to Jamaica and Brazil, we have political, militia and police

---

1   www.stonewall.org.uk/sites/default/files/lgbt_in_britain_home_and_communities. pdf
2   https://transequality.org/blog/murders-of-transgender-people-in-2020-surpasses-total-for-last-year-in-just-seven-months

groups rounding up the queers, killing, maiming or imprisoning them. In some parts of the world, to get access to gender affirming surgeries or therapies, trans people must still be sterilized, by law.[3]

We've got people in Boston marching for Straight Pride, calls for our existence to be silent and preferably invisible, unless, of course, it's for their entertainment or pornography. We are to be accused of 'shoving it down people's throats'. We've only recently had our kisses, stories and lives represented in films, TV shows, government and sport. We have only been able to get married since 2000 (initially in the Netherlands, followed by just another 26 countries over the next 19 years).

This is a world where a court defence will hear and be influenced by the 'Gay Panic' defence,[4] where juries have been deadlocked on a murder case purely because the sexual orientation or the gender assigned at birth of a person was, according to the defendant, discovered after sex and the murderer was so enraged by the 'discovery' that they pleaded that this is a reasonable explanation as to why they murdered them.

We aren't just caricatures of flamboyant, catty men or butch, aggressive women. We exist in an endless myriad of existences. We are other than what the world expects or defaults to (straight, cisgender, white, non-disabled, housed etc.).

We thank our elders, across counties, races and religions, for their tireless and life-costing work they have done so far, but we are far from finished. We are far from equality.

We are here, we are queer, we procreate.

Get used to it.

Why?

This book is a chance to broaden your understanding and ability to support those who birth and parent beyond the binary, and the world's cis heteronormative.

---

3   www.nbcnews.com/feature/nbc-out/japan-s-supreme-court-upholds-transgender-sterilization-requirement-n962721

4   www.americanbar.org/groups/crsj/publications/member-features/gay-trans-panic-defense

It is not the end, the final word on everything you will ever need to know. It's the start of your journey to being LGBT+ competent. Keep moving forward, keep talking, but know when to shush and listen, watch and absorb. Learn when to elevate the work of others, and when and how to speak up if it feels wrong.

Parts of this book have been written by individuals with first-hand experience of the oppression and difficulties of birthing, parenting or working in the industry's cis heteronormative bubble. Parts that aren't written by the author directly are credited with the individual's information and contact details. When seeking information or education it is best to go directly to that community to listen and learn. However, take time to consider the emotional labour you are asking others to spend on your education. Payment has been made to everyone who has shared their time and story with us. We should never expect to be given this knowledge or skills for nothing.

Due to the very nature of the LGBT+ community, it is forever changing. Folk are always finding their people, finding their specific place on the spectrum of sexuality and gender. The infinite differences are important. They enable alienated folks who feel wrong or broken to find others who feel the same. Finding someone to walk the back streets of your mind and feelings with is a joy, a validation that cannot be underestimated. The alternative is that we have 11-year-olds typing 'Why do I like girls and boys?' into BBC Bitesize because they are genuinely convinced that they are broken (showing my age here with BBC Bitesize!). We must never lose sight of the fact that although our differences are important, they do not divide the unity of our shared othering from the world's cis heteronormativity.

As the title of this book suggests, because we have babies, we parent, we feed our babies. We want or need access to services and products. The difficulty comes when providers are worried about saying the wrong thing, so they say nothing at all. So, this is one of the aims of this book – to hold the hands of professionals on those first few tentative steps into the inclusion of queerness.

Queer people walk through the world differently. We are treated differently, we are the other, an asterisk or an afterthought. We are asked if our wives are our mothers, sisters, friends before the thought occurs that they could be our spouse. We are asked where the mother is when we try to access maternity units during labour. We are asked who the 'real' mother is, who the 'real' father is, and we are asked what is 'going on...down there'. We are othered.

My role in the book is to be a doula for you through the process. To walk alongside you and point out interesting and important aspects as you read.

It might be helpful to have a paper and pen with you to jot down questions you have about the services you provide, the questions you may want to ask your National Health Service (NHS) trust regarding their policies and processes that might put LGBT+ families at risk of falling through the cracks.

Silence is deafening. If you want to include and serve LGBT+ people then stand up and be seen as an ally. Filling your feed with thin, white, cis, hetero, two-parent families will attract those families, but if you believe that everyone deserves the support and services that you offer, take a deep breath. Read on.

CHAPTER 1

Alphabet Soup

LGBTQQIAP

Let's strip this back.

Please use the definitions below as a generalization. We are only able to use the language that we have at the time. Not every single person will fit neatly into these generalizations. Some people you will meet and have an expectation of who they are or who they love based on their label, but this won't always be correct. Remember not to centre your expectation. Instead, centring the person telling you who they are is allyship 101. Being able to separate your expectation from their reality is essential. The most important thing to remember is simply that people are who they say they are. No one has a right to dictate or allow any identification.

Lesbian: A woman who is attracted to women. The common misconception with lesbians is that they are women who sleep with other women. There are a couple reasons why we should avoid qualifying anyone's sexuality with who they have sex with. When we have a tick list in our minds of what qualifies someone to call themselves something, we are an active participant in gatekeeping, or keeping people out of an identity based on our list or expectation. This is often expressed as 'How do you know you are a lesbian if you haven't slept with a woman?' or 'Maybe you just haven't found the right man!' Another problem with quantifying particularly women and those assigned female at birth with who they have or haven't had sex with is that it furthers the overt sexualization of women and those assigned female at birth. Who are constantly in the most searched lists on pornography websites? The LGBT+ community is overtly sexualized, everything we do is seen as sexual – holding hands with our partners is seen as sexualized, not for children's eyes, not in public, for goodness sake! A government survey in 2018 found that two-thirds of LGBT+ people feel uncomfortable holding hands in public.[1] Even in 2019, in a metropolitan city like London, lesbians were attacked simply for not complying with kissing on the orders of men aged 15–18. For all LGBT+ people, our identities are often reduced to either the flamboyant or aggressive characters we are so often portrayed as in books and on the screen, or we are reduced purely to sex, who we do or don't have it with.

Gay: A man who is attracted to men. As with lesbians, gay men are often reduced to men who have sex with men, removing the love, the relationship, the people. Gay can also be a catch-all term for the LGBT+ communities: gay night at the local night club, gay Pride, gay marriage and so on. You will more often find Pride events being called after the city, so Mancheter Pride, Brighton Pride, rather than simply Gay Pride. The laws in the UK have always focused on homosexuality. Homosexual sex was illegal in England and Wales until 1967,[2] until 1980 in Scotland and 1982 in Northern Ireland. The Sexual Offences Act of 1967 was updated to make consenting sex legal between two men, aged over 21, in private. Prosecutions for relationships between two consenting men over the age of 16 continued until the new millennium, when the age of consent was equalized.[3] We see where the attitude of 'whatever two consenting adults get up to in their own homes, in private, is up to them!' comes from. As recently as 2013, a law was passed pardoning gay men previously convicted of offences.[4] It was dubbed 'Turing's Law' after Alan Turing, the British

---

1   https://assets.publishing.service.gov.uk/government/uploads/system/uploads/attachment_data/file/722314/GEO-LGBT-Survey-Report.pdf

2   www.legislation.gov.uk/ukpga/1967/60/pdfs/ukpga_19670060_en.pdf

3   www.legislation.gov.uk/ukpga/2000/44/contents

4   www.gov.uk/government/news/thousands-officially-pardoned-under-turings-law

mathematician and computer scientist famous for his role in breaking Nazi ciphers during World War 2. Turing was convicted in 1952 of homosexual acts and accepted chemical castration as treatment for his offence. He died two years later from cyanide poisoning, which was ruled as suicide. This was just over half a century ago, in the UK. Not a long, long time ago, in a galaxy far, far away. This happened here, in a time where some of us were alive. If we weren't, our elders certainly were.

Bisexual: Someone attracted to their own and other genders and/or sex. In 2015, a YouGov survey asked people to plot themselves on a 'sexuality scale', one end being 'exclusively heterosexual' and the other being 'exclusively homosexual'. Forty-nine per cent of 18–24-year-olds chose something other than completely heterosexual.

Figure 1.1: British adults place themselves on the Kinsey Scale, ranging from 0 (completely heterosexual) to 6 (completely homosexual)

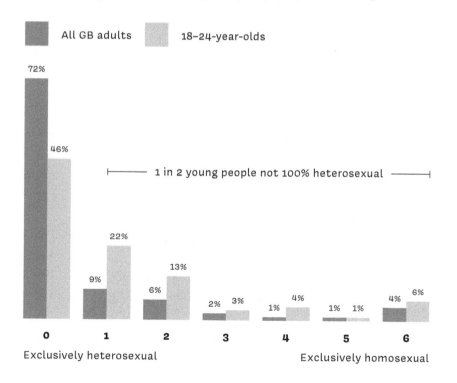

Figure 1.2: Across generations

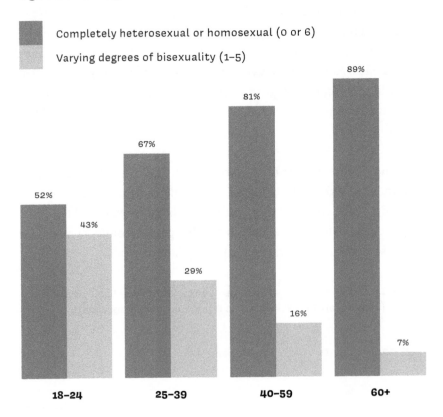

Completely heterosexual or homosexual (0 or 6)

Varying degrees of bisexuality (1–5)

Forty-six per cent of 18–24-year-olds are at the exclusively hetero-sexual end and six per cent are exclusively homosexual.

Those in the 1–6 ranges on this chart aren't exclusively heterosexual. People who ticked 1–6 in the 18–24-year-old category make up 49 per cent of the population.[5]

With each generation, we see a falling in folk identifying as binary sexualities: heterosexual and homosexual.

The charts help us to examine the age-old assumption that bisex-ual people are 50 per cent straight, and 50 per cent gay. Bisexuality

---

5   https://yougov.co.uk/topics/lifestyle/articles-reports/2015/08/16/half-young-not-heterosexual

exists as a spectrum. If you exist outside the exclusively straight or gay camps, at whichever point along this spectrum and wish to identify as bisexual, then you are bisexual.

As with all LGBT+ people, bisexuals are questioned or asked to justify their identity, particularly if they are currently with a different sex partner. If bisexuals are with a same-sex partner, then the world assumes that they are gay. Bisexuals are frequently erased in studies and data collection. They made up nearly half of the 18–24-year-olds in 2015, yet, here we still are, arguing with the world whether bisexuality is valid.

Transgender: A person whose gender differs from their assigned sex at birth. A common misconception is that transgender or trans means to transition, from male to female or female to male. Again, we must look at our gatekeeping assumptions. We must understand that there are no qualifying criteria which enable or bar a person from identifying as trans. A person who obtains a gender recognition certificate (GRC), legally changing their gender, is no more trans than someone who does not. Someone who has surgery, cuts their hair, changes their name, takes hormones and so on is no more trans than someone who doesn't want or need to take those steps.

Since the Gender Recognition Act was introduced in 2004, trans people have been able to apply for a GRC. The GRC process in the UK currently requires: two doctors to diagnose the person with gender dysphoria, a £5 fee payable to the Gender Recognition Panel (GRP), the signed consent of their spouse, if they are married, and them to have lived in their acquired identity for at least two years.

The GRP, which consists of legal and medical people, will then assess the application and either grant or deny it.

The Equality Act 2010 protects against discrimination based on gender reassignment[6] – anyone who is proposing, undergoing or has undergone the process (or part of the process) for the purpose of reassigning the person's sex. Non-binary people may or may not

---

6   www.legislation.gov.uk/ukpga/2010/15/section/7

identify as transgender, given that their gender does not match the one assigned at birth. More on non-binary folk later.

Queer: Someone who isn't cis or straight. Queer has its roots in oppression. Queer bashing was a thing, and indeed still is. Queer is still used today as a slur. It is still hurled at LGBT+ persons, and non-LGBT+ persons when the aggressor has decided they might be LGBT+. Some LGBT+ folk want to reclaim this word and wear it proudly as a badge of honour, an act of defiance against the past and current offenders of hate crimes. Some people within the LGBT+ community do not want to be called queer, and again we must remember that it is not up to anyone but the person themselves to choose the words that they use to describe themselves.

Questioning: Someone who knows they aren't cis and/or heterosexual but hasn't found their space on the spectrum yet. They may not want to find it or they may be searching – either is valid. Questioning is often seen as a stopover on route to the person's 'true' identity. Some people are happy to be here, this is their destination. They are questioning the worlds of cis heteronormality and they are happy to be here.

Intersex: A general term used for a variety of conditions which mean a person's sexual or reproductive anatomy, hormones or chromosomes that don't fit the typical definitions of the sex binary. Intersex people exist in a variety of bodies. There is no standard intersex condition. It can be visible at birth, or it can be invisible and discovered later in life, or never known. Roughly 1 in 1500 people are born with an intersex condition,[7] which makes it as common as people born with ginger hair. We are expected, by western society, to fit neatly into two boxes, male or female. Sexuality is a spectrum, as recently evidenced by the YouGov poll on sexuality mentioned earlier; gender is a spectrum, and sex can be too.

---

7   https://isna.org/faq/frequency

Asexual: This is almost impossible to sum up in a succinct sentence. Asexual people may fall in love, want a relationship, experience sexual desire, choose to masturbate, choose to engage in sexual activity, and some may not. What asexuality isn't is abstinence, sexual repression, dysfunction, or a lack of libido due to circumstance. A very common and tiresome use of the term is: 'I was a bit asexual for a while when I had my baby.'

Western society expects people to have sex. A lot if not nearly all motives of people are expected to be governed by sexual desire and the pursuit of sex. Again, consider gatekeeping in your own assumption of asexuality.

Pansexual: Someone who is attracted to people regardless of their gender/sex/identification. Bisexuality and pansexuality are often confused. They are not the same. They are not interchangeable or synonyms. A frequently held belief is that bisexual means two – men and women – and that therefore pansexual means any. This notion is incorrect and is biphobic. Bisexuals are not trans exclusionary. The differences may seem small and very nuanced, but they are very important to some people, so, again, simply respect the information that the person you are talking to gives you and don't second guess or make assumptions based on their identity.

Cis: Not trans. In a world where trans people are at a higher risk of physical, emotional and financial mistreatment, we must understand the importance of not 'othering' minorities or oppressed people. If we use 'woman' and 'trans woman', what we are really saying here is that trans woman is 'other'. This is a not-so-subtle way to signal to your audience that woman means woman and trans woman means what exactly? There will be occasions where it is necessary to distinguish them, for example in a medical scenario. It may be imperative to know a cis woman, a trans man and an assigned female at birth (AFAB) non-binary person will have different medical needs and want to be offered different screenings (like cervical smears) from a cis man, trans woman and those assigned male at birth (AMAB). By using cis woman and trans woman, we aren't singling out either group. We aren't forcing the minority into a smaller box with an asterisk or explanation next to their name. The cis community is shouldering some of the burden, so to speak. That's how you show allyship.

Non-binary: The simplest explanation is the transgender explanation, that your sex assigned at birth doesn't match your gender. Non-binary folk can be AFAB or AMAB. Non-binary people may be intersex. Non-binary is valid as a standalone identification or gender, but it isn't a 'straight' swap from male to female, for example.

Non-binary folks will look, think and feel a variety of different ways; there is no queer uniform that we must wear to be non-binary. It is important to remember that not everyone wants to change their body, the way they walk, the way they talk, but just know that they don't fit the binary (man or woman). Non-binary folks do not owe the world androgyny.

There is currently no legal status or gender marker that a non-binary person can apply or be given in the UK. Some countries such as Australia, India and Canada, and some states in the USA, have an opt-in third gender option on documents.[8] Some countries have an option for an opt-in for intersex people only. Several attempts have been made in UK parliament to have a third gender marker available for non-binary or gender non-confirming people, but as yet, none have been successful.

You may hear people say that trans rights are 30–40 years behind the rights of LGB people. This is because although homosexuality was decriminalized in the 1960s, it wasn't until the new millennium that trans binary people were able to apply for a gender recognition certificate, or legally be able to change their gender. So, the gap between non-binary rights and the rights of LGB people is still growing. We are still unable to legally exist. When that will be continues to feel further and further away. Attempts were made in 2015 and 2018 to have the UK government recognize a third gender option for people.

---

8   www.pinknews.co.uk/2019/07/14/non-binary-rights-countries-better-than-uk

The Gender Recognition Act reform 2017–18 saw that over half (58.2%) of people responding to the survey agreed that there needs to be changes to the GRC to accommodate individuals who identify as non-binary.[9]

Despite the results of the Gender Recognition Act reform survey being overwhelmingly in favour of reforming the act, making the process simpler for trans binary people, and inclusive of non-binary people, the government declined to act on the results.

Ally: Sometimes you may see an extra A in the LGBTQIAA acronym. This is often depicted as ally – someone who is straight or cis and stands with LGBT+ people. We love you; we need you, but this isn't what the A stands for. If you are an ally, or an aspiring ally, then this is your first exercise in learning and remembering to stop centring cis heteronormality in your world.

Womxn: I get asked this one a lot. Often, I see people use womxn to add in non-binary people assigned female at birth and trans women into women. Non-binary people regardless of their assigned sex at birth aren't women. Trans women are women, so why do we need to use womxn?

Pronouns: These can include:

- He/him/his
- She/her/hers
- They/them/theirs
- Ze/zem/zirs.

This is not an exhaustive list by any means, but these may be the ones that you are most likely to hear. Pronouns also don't equal gender. Just because someone uses they/them pronouns it doesn't mean that they are non-binary, for example.

---

9 https://commonslibrary.parliament.uk/research-briefings/cbp-9079

Gender neutral pronouns: Often, I am told 'I can't refer to you as they/them as it's a plural'. To this I say that when we sit down at a table and see a phone left from the previous occupier we say, 'Oh no! Someone left their phone, I'll hand it in in case they come back for it.' Or if someone says, 'Oh, my cousin is in the hospital', we might say, 'Oh, that's terrible, I hope they are okay.'

Some sources date this language back to the 14th century; however, we know that two spirit people have existed for centuries in First Nations and Indigenous communities in North America.[10] Other trans and non-binary identities existed across the globe long before colonization and the insistence of the gender binary came along.

Even if, just for a second, we pretend that gender neutral pronouns are grammatically incorrect (even though we know they're not), does the need to be grammatically correct come before the right of the person in question to be safe, loved and valid? We know that using chosen names and pronouns dramatically reduces the risk of suicide. The *Journal of Adolescent Health* in 2018 published research showing that using a person's chosen name and pronouns may cut the risk of suicide by a massive 65 per cent.[11] Hardly a comparison, is it?

Titles can include: Mrs, Ms, Miss, Mx (pronounced Mix), Mr.

Passing/Clocky: The trans community sometimes uses these two opposing terms to describe whether a person 'passes' as cisgender. Can they walk down the street without being 'clocked' as being trans?

Passing isn't always the aim for trans folks. Many don't want to pass, but some do as a matter of safety, and not just in bad neighbourhoods or alleyways at the dead of night. Trans folks have been attacked in broad daylight.

Closeted/Outed: This describes someone not 'out' as their sexuality or gender identification, for a variety of reasons, often but not exclusively limited to their own emotional or physical safety. Those who remain

---

10   https://lgbtqhealth.ca/community/two-spirit.php
11   https://pubmed.ncbi.nlm.nih.gov/29609917

closeted should never be forced to be out or be 'outed' by anyone. Letting slip that a service user is queer when they aren't out can have huge implications for their safety and their life. Their reasons are their own, and you cannot presume their status, or what is best for them.

Drag kings and queens: Drag is a performance, often over the top, beautiful and expressive versions of femininity and masculinity. Drag isn't a synonym for trans. Drag kings and queens may be trans, but they may also be cis and don their drag persona for performance only.

'T' and 'E': Testosterone and oestrogen. Folk may want to or choose to take hormones – hormone replacement therapy (HRT) – to change their bodies to closer fit their identity. You may hear someone say 'I've been on T for two years now' or 'It's my T-anniversary'. More on hormones later.

Theybie: Some parents, regardless of sexuality or gender identity, may choose to raise their children as gender neutral. This means that they won't use gendered pronouns for their baby. They may use they/them for their babies' pronouns. Study after study have shown that assigning a baby a gender different from their sex means that adults and others will interact with them differently.[12] Many parents feel that giving the babies they perceive as boys toys that seek to aid development in building, and giving the babies they perceive as girls dollies and toys that aim to develop speech and caring skills, is unnecessary and will restrict the opportunities for education and learning of life skills for their child.

Gender affirming surgeries: 'Have you had *the* surgery?' This is a question that gender queer people get asked often. There is not *one* surgery that gender queer people have. Some folks don't want any – this doesn't make them less trans.

---

12   www.apa.org/pubs/journals/releases/bne-bne0000199.pdf

Top surgery: This could include:

- Chest reconstruction – an AFAB person's chest/breast is reconstructed to have the appearance of larger pectoral muscles associated with AMAB people.
- Bottom surgery:

    - vaginoplasty, where an AMAB person undertakes major surgery to remove and reconstruct their genitals
    - labiaplasty, which involves the creation or augmentation of labia (some cis people have labiaplasty too. They may want to change the physical appearance of their labia)
    - penectomy: removal of the penis
    - orchiectomy: removal of the testicles.

- Voice surgery – augmentation of the vocal cords to deeper or raise the natural pitch of the person's voice.
- Face and neck surgery: this can include shaving or the removal of bones or plates to give a more feminine or masculine appearance.

Dysphoria: The 'disconnect' a person feels about the body they are in, to their identity. Not all gender queer folks experience dysphoria, and what one person experiences as dysphoric another may find euphoric. There is no right or wrong. Common sources of dysphoria include: voice, size or shape of breast/chest, hip size/shape ('childbearing hips'), as well as non-physical traits like gait or walk, mannerisms.

Dysphoria can also come from the outside world. You can be loving living in your body, with all its parts and aspects; however, the way the world treats you because of your body could be a source of dysphoria.

Misgendering/Dead-naming: To call a person the pronouns given to their gender assigned at birth or the name given to them at birth rather than their chosen name. Research published in 2018 in the *Journal of Adolescent Health* revealed that using a person's chosen name and pronouns may cut the risk of suicide by a massive 65 per cent.[13] Given that research by Stonewall has uncovered that a staggering 89 per cent of trans people have considered suicide, and 27 per cent have attempted suicide,[14] using their chosen name and pronouns isn't just polite, it could be a matter of life and death.

Chest-feeding: Some gender queer folks may want to refer to feeding their babies with their bodies as chest-feeding to avoid dysphoria at the assumed femininity of the term breast. We all have breast tissues, and cis men can get breast cancer, but it's not up to anyone other than the person in question as to how they want their bodies to be referred to. Some folks may also use nurse or suckle. My favourite is stillen, a German word which has many translations: to quiet, to comfort, suckle, satisfy, nurse, stop, still, quench. This also serves a purpose to understand that breast- or chest-feeding is not just about transfer of calories. A baby doesn't ask to go to the breast/chest purely for calories. They ask for a huge variety of reasons. They may ask because they are cold, and the arms of their parent provide warmth. They may be frightened, and the closeness of their parent provides comfort and calm. They may be asking their parent to slow down, take time with them, look at them, bond with them. (More about inducing lactation later.)

---

13   www.apa.org/pubs/journals/releases/bne-bne0000199.pdf
14   www.stonewall.org.uk/system/files/lgbt_in_britain_health.pdf

CHAPTER 2

Language, Assumptions, Delivery

Now that we have a basic understanding of some terminology and language let's look at what I believe are the three main barriers for LGBT+ parents.

1. Language

2. Assumptions

3. Delivery

In most of the examples of LGBT+ parents being at increased physical or emotional risk, alienation or erasure, we can see at least one of these barriers being a contributing factor.

Language

Language doesn't just mean the language that you speak. It includes that language on your forms and your signage. The language on your social media. If you are a birth worker who uses social media – as most of us do – then how will LGBT+ parents know that you have considered them? That you welcome them? That you want to care for them? If language that affirms us is missing? If you work for a wider company or collective, are they going to look at your organization's page to find you on a directory or such like, and what are they going to see there? If you work for the NHS, do LGBT+ parents have a box on your forms where they can be recorded? Non-gestational mothers for example. Does your NHS trust have any masculine language maternity notes? Or any gender-neutral ones? Brighton & Sussex NHS Trust has these forms available for those who need them. Could your trust do this? We will speak to a midwife from Brighton & Sussex University Hospital later to find out what this looks like in practice.

It is not as simple as removing the word woman and putting in parent. If we were to do this with some procedures and protections, for example the process of abortion in the UK, could changing this language lead to a situation where non-gestational parents can soon ask for an abortion?

The rights for women have been fought for with literal blood, sweat and tears. We cannot risk any roll back or dilution. I am a champion for additive language. We can add to language to ensure that more people are included.

The current wording of the Equality Act of 2010[1] states that it is discrimination to treat a woman unfavourably because she is breast-feeding. Would a trans man with a gender recognition certificate be covered? To my knowledge this hasn't been tested but it begs the question of what other protections trans men may be missing out on. Protection against pregnancy-related dismissal, maternity/paternity pay, to make reasonable adjustments for him...the list goes on. Scotland did make a change that removes the word woman, but in doing so has cast the net wider to include more people. The Breastfeeding etc. (Scotland) Act of 2005 states that it is an offence to deliberately prevent or stop a person in charge of a child from feeding milk to that child in public.[2] This change has widened the net to include bot-tle-feeding parents, chest-feeding parents, co-nursing parents, trans men, non-binary people and those who are finger feeding, syringe feeding, cup feeding, SNS (supplemental nursing system) feeding or tube feeding. The change also ensures that the rights of the child are the focus. The child's right to be fed when they are hungry is at the

---

1   https://assets.publishing.service.gov.uk/government/uploads/system/uploads/attachment_data/file/85008/business-quickstart.pdf
2   www.legislation.gov.uk/asp/2005/1/pdfs/asp_20050001_en.pdf

forefront. However, who is giving the milk is protected because it is the child's right to be fed when they need to be.

Just as LGBT+ parents should have the right to see language that reflects them, women and mothers also have that right. We cannot go forwards by going backwards.

Some businesses may exist purely to serve LGBT+ parents, or specifically gender queer folk. They may choose to not include any language relating to mothers or women. That is their choice in their business policy. Similarly, companies, collectives and individuals who don't wish to support queer folk also have that choice. However, we cannot claim to support all parents if we mean cisgender, heterosexual women. If we put a barrier on to who we support, who we reflect in our language, we cannot be miffed when LGBT+ parents and our allies don't consider it to be inclusive.

In the birthing world, we talk about language a lot. Hypnobirthing talks about surges rather than contractions, power rather than pain; language is an important and intrinsic part of our world.

Midwives in the UK are moving away from using 'delivered' to mean the baby has been born. When I spoke to a community midwife at a home birth in London during the winter of 2018, when the family's baby was born before her arrival (commonly known as birth before arrival, BBA), the midwife asked me how many babies I had 'delivered'. I told her I had birthed two, and this was the first time I had had to catch a baby. (Doulas don't do this as standard, as we are not medical professionals. We only intervene if harm will come if we don't.) When the second midwife arrived 20 minutes or so after the baby was born, the first midwife recalled our conversation, and the second midwife said, 'Oh yes, we aren't meant to say delivered anymore. You used to have to do X amount of deliveries, but now we are meant to say "catches".' Babies aren't pizza. They aren't delivered, they are born – whether that's at home with twinkly lights and a slightly soggy-shoed but safe-handed doula, or in an operating theatre. Babies are born.

Language, as many scholars have tried to deduce over the years, speaks to our history and our future. Often, we see headlines expressing outrage about new words being added to our dictionary and our everyday lexicon. As a product of the late 1980s, early 90s, I grew up texting, and this brings its own language, like emojis. I remember seeing a *Tomorrow's World* snippet – I imagine it was the mid to late 90s – explaining to people what an emoji was. Back then it was a semi-colon and an open or closed bracket to decree emotion. Now we've got aubergines and peaches.

Language is forever changing, in the birth and wider world, it matters. It is what separates us, what brings us together. For most queer folk, it is important.

As previously discussed, we know that using the correct pronouns and chosen name reduces the risk of suicide among trans and non-binary youth. Explaining to cis folk how it feels to be misgendered or dead-named is difficult. When you are misgendering folks, for example using he/him pronouns for a trans woman who has told you her pronouns are she/her, what you are really saying is 'I don't believe you'. When you call a trans man her, what you are saying is 'You are wrong, I am right'. When you gender a non-binary person, you are saying 'My need to be "right" is more important than your safety and emotional wellbeing'.

We must then consider the impact of healthcare professionals using the 'incorrect' language (pronouns and so on) during the pregnancy journey.

Being misgendered or dead-named by your healthcare professional can be catastrophic for the trust and bond that should be building during this most vulnerable time. Having a healthcare professional out us to an entire ward or waiting room, for example, would no doubt trigger our fight or flight response. We would know that the treatment we could receive from the public as well as the healthcare professional themselves could be a risk. This fight or flight response will kick-start our adrenaline, which shuts down the body's ability to make oxytocin. We need oxytocin, sometimes known as the 'love hormone', for many things in our lives, including breast-/chest-feeding and birth.

We know that for our bodies to birth effectively we need to feel safe, above all else. When I get calls from a family who are 'overdue',[3] parents sometimes want ideas for 'natural' ways to bring their baby earth side. Natural induction is a bit of an oxymoron. One way to encourage birth is to induce oxytocin. This might be sex or masturbation, laughing your head off to a funny film or eating your favourite food. So, we know oxytocin is essential for birth, but not feeling loved, respected and safe means no oxytocin. See where I am going?

If we are worried or scared, our labour can stop or delay. It can lengthen our labour, increasing the risk of intervention, which, in turn, increases the risk of further intervention. This could mean further risk, further intervention, and on and on the cascade of intervention goes.

This is where we get to the nitty gritty. Should we just call people ovary vessels and penis holders so that everyone is clear up front what biological functions they may or may not have?

I don't believe that the erasure of gendered language is necessary for everyone to be able to access support. We might be using a few more words than before, we might have to edit our forms and move things about, maybe change the font size to get everything in, but can we put the price of ink ahead of the price of inclusion?

Think about the number of forms you have to fill out in a year of your life. Think about the amount that your service users had to fill in the year of their pregnancy and birth of their baby. Its endless paperwork. Tick boxes for Mother, Father, Male, Female, Relationship to child (please tick Woman/Mother). I am still to be convinced that it's for the betterment of birth that Woman or Mother should be removed entirely. It's incredibly important that credit is given where it is due to most people who birth all the babies in the world: the mothers, the women. However, we must be careful that we acknowledge that not all who go through a birth are women.

When we look at the laws in the UK, anyone who gives birth is

---

3   A pet hate of mine is the term 'overdue'. Babies aren't buses (see earlier regarding delivery: babies aren't pizza). Term for an average pregnancy is 36–42 weeks; a due date is the date 40 weeks from the last menstrual cycle, thus it is ridiculous to hold it in such high esteem for deciding when babies should be born.

recorded as the mother.[4] At the time of writing there is an ongoing legal battle for a trans man, Freddy McConnell, to be recorded as the father of his baby.[5] Being recorded as a mother on an official document when you are a man will trigger the dysphoria monster. Plus, it isn't accurate! It brings a grey area to the GRC (gender recognition certificate). Having legally obtained a GRC, this father is legally a man, and yet also the mother. Many people will be awaiting the outcome of this appeal with bated breath. Some countries do allow for transgender parents to be recorded as parent.[6]

Non-binary parents will also be waiting for the outcome of Freddy's appeal. Non-binary parents, just like this father, will be recorded incorrectly as the mother, or the father, if they are the non-gestational parent. There is currently no legal document like the GRC that non-binary folks can obtain to prove their gender, or lack thereof. However, if permission is granted for Freddy to be recorded as the father, as some same-sex couples will be recorded, then perhaps there is hope for non-binary parents to be afforded the same options.[7]

Since 2003,[8] some counties have been issuing documents like driving licences and passports with a 'third' option for gender, usually an 'X'. We know that two spirit people existed centuries ago, in the First Nation and Indigenous peoples of North America, so it's hardly new-fangled ideology that gender existing only as a binary is too ridged to hold us all.

Back in the modern-day UK, trans men with GRCs may not be able to access the information or protections of the Equality Act 2010. The Act states that it is discrimination to a 'woman' to 'treat her unfavourably because of a pregnancy of hers'.[9] It also states that it is discrimination to 'treat a woman unfavourably because she is

4   www.legislation.gov.uk/ukpga/2008/22/contents
5   www.theguardian.com/society/2020/nov/16/trans-man-loses-uk-legal-battle-to-register-as-his-childs-father
6   https://tgeu.org/council-of-europe-recognises-trans-parents
7   www.gov.uk/register-birth/who-can-register-a-birth
8   https://ihra.org.au/21597/ten-years-of-x-passports-and-no-protection-from-discrimination
9   www.legislation.gov.uk/ukpga/2010/15/section/18

breastfeeding'. We see how quickly the waters can become 'muddied', with queer folks and their babies slipping through the net of protection.

As previously discussed, the Scottish Government has found a way to cut through the confusion to ensure that parents, caregivers, aunts, uncles, whoever is 'in charge' of a baby (although, in my experience, it's usually the baby that is in charge) can feed their baby milk in public. Scotland's Breastfeeding etc. Act states[10] 'it is an offence deliberately to prevent or stop a person in charge of a child from feeding milk to that child in a public place or on licensed premises'. The wording of this legislation is my go-to example of how we can protect everyone's right to feed their babies. Breast- and chest-feeding will always likely draw more negative attention in public than bottle feeding, as bottle feeding is often perceived as the norm in western society. However, this legislation doesn't exclude anyone from the right to feed their baby milk, be that by bottled formula, expressed breast milk, tube fed, SNS feeding (more on this later), finger feeding or any other of the incredible ways that we give nourishment to our children. Wherever, whoever, you are allowed, you are protected – one point for Scotland.

Removing the words woman and mother is also not a variable option. If we were to remove 'woman' from all documents and legislations currently in place to protect them against obstetric or other violence when giving birth, with say 'parent', we would open the possibility of the partner of the gestational parent or woman giving birth making decisions about their pregnancy. This might include how or where to give birth for example. As a doula, I have been in consultant appointments where doctors have turned to fathers and asked for permission to do a 'sweep'. A sweep is a medical procedure that might be offered in the later stages of pregnancy, where a midwife or obstetrician will use their fingers to 'sweep' the membranes of the baby's sack away from the walls of the uterus in a bid to induce labour – a very common but little discussed procedure in pregnancy that, despite popular belief, does carry risks.

---

10   www.legislation.gov.uk/asp/2005/1/pdfs/asp_20050001_en.pdf

So, if in the legislation we used parent for example rather than mother, or pregnant woman, this could open these and other choices surrounding body autonomy to being accessible by the non-gestational parent. I have seen papers for caesarean sections be signed by fathers and husbands, and I know of at least one set that were signed by the baby's grandparent. We cannot risk these sparse and under-enforced and little understood rights of body autonomy being diluted. That does not mean we cannot add to the language. The policy could read 'All mothers and birthing parents can be offered a sweep at 40 weeks of gestation' rather than 'All parents should be offered a sweep at 40 weeks of gestation'. Changing the wording to 'parents should be offered a sweep' could mean that non-gestational parents have a say on the gestational parent's body autonomy – having a sweep, or not having a sweep – but if we ensure that the mother, the gestational parent, is the focus of all choices, it will ensure that they have full autonomy at all times.

Another example I like to use is that we often must go back and retrofit accessibility equipment when we realize that it is no longer serving as many people as possible. Historical buildings have been fitted with ramps and lifts, and as the child of an amputee paraplegic, I notice the ramps! Centuries-old castles have been fitted with hearing loops for the hearing impaired. Toilets are starting to be upgraded to changing spaces so that older/heavier children and people can be safely changed in public. These changes aren't coming quickly enough and are not as widespread as they could be mind you, but I still do a mini whoop each time I notice an accessible changing space.

The point is, when a product or service is no longer working for a society, we should and can make changes, go back and add, reword, rework how the space or service works, try and make it as accessible as possible. Ramps on the steps of the Natural History Museum take nothing away from the hundreds of thousands of non-disabled visitors every year, but they make it a damn sight easier for more people to access the building.

When I state that we routinely ask loads of people for their preferred names, this is normally met by scoffs and confused looks, until I talk about grandparents. In my immediate family alone we have Grandad, Grumpsy, Grandpops, Nanny, Grandma, Grapsey (the smallest couldn't say Great Nanny, so it was Grapes Nanny, Grapes and now Grapsey – cute, right?).

So, when I meet grandparents in settings from Sling Library meets, to postnatal doula support meetings, I simply ask, 'What are you going to go by?' There is no nervousness or offence on either side. It is just a question. If we can do this unconsciously, and in complete acceptance of the respondent's choice, we can take steps to do that with LGBT+ parents too.

Many same-sex parents will work with variations on the 'norm' of Mum, Mummy, Mama, Dad, Daddy, Papa. Non-binary parents may use Bubba, Moddy – a mix of Mom and Dad – Zaza and more.

The point is that we never shout down a grandma arguing that 'my grandmother was always called Nanny so I will be called Nanny!' We accept, adapt our language, and move on. In a similar way when our friend gets married, we might slip up because we've said their maiden name for decades and that unconscious assumption will take some conscious unlearning, but we will get there. If we want to. We don't insist on using their previous name, if of course they have chosen to change their name after getting married.

Cis heteronormality will not disappear overnight if we take steps to include more people in our thoughts and hearts when talking about, providing services and designing products for people who birth and parent their babies.

Assumptions

We all make assumptions. It can be a real timesaver. The trouble comes when the assumption from the system or the individual within that system is that everyone accessing that system or service will be cisgender and heterosexual. An example of this is creating pathways for funding for sperm donation on the NHS that exclude same-sex couples.

It is very possible that the next person who comes to your clinic or contacts you regarding your services could be an LGBT+ parent.

With time, that likelihood is only going to increase, as we know more and more people with every generation identify as something other than exclusively heterosexual (see Chapter 1).

The systems, pathways and referral criteria were all made for and by cis heteronormality. Have they ever been updated with LGBT+ parents specifically in mind?

In Chapter 8, We Actually Exist, we will see more examples how the assumption of who needs these services or products not only unfairly restricts and excludes LGBT+ parents but could and has increased the risk for them and their babies.

Even if we move past the assumptions relating to access and visibility of LGBT+ parents then we must still talk about the assumptions of unconscious biases we hold relating to LGBT+ people. Are these unconscious biases leaking into our business, leaking into how we care for people?

We know that unconscious bias affects the treatment that black and brown mothers and parents receive in the maternity system in the UK. The MBRRACE[11] report tells us that black mothers are five times more likely to die than white mothers. Asian mothers are three times more likely to die. The reason is not that black and brown bodies are broken, wrong or less than other bodies. It is largely due to the conscious and unconscious bias of the system and the individual. This is further evidenced by the fact that, in the US, black babies are three times more likely to die in hospital than white newborn babies. This disparity halves when black babies are cared for by a black doctor.[12] Unconscious bias also means that women and pregnant people who cover their heads (Muslim, Jewish, Orthodox Christian etc.) also wait longer for pain relief than their non-covered counterparts. We all have unconscious bias. Whether this is viewed as a 'good' or 'bad' bias, we must acknowledge that not discussing or dismantling our bias is killing people.

Unconscious bias seeps into everything we do as human beings;

---

11   www.npeu.ox.ac.uk/mbrrace-uk
12   www.bmj.com/content/370/bmj.m3315

we all have bias. Undertaking training to identify and assess your unconscious biases is the first step to improving outcomes for those who birth outside your 'norm'.

Delivery

Having all the language down, examining the assumptions that you make as a person and the assumptions that your NHS trust or business makes about the people it may serve, is kind of pointless until you are able to deliver the changes needed.

If the next person to come to you in need of your help is part of a same-sex couple, a non-binary person or a trans person, how prepared are you? You've done the background work, you've improved and added to your language, you've done the work internally and are now, at least, aware of your bias and how that may affect the care you give or the way that the person in front of you can move through the system. What now?

Start small if you are worried. Practise giving your pronouns and asking for them from people in passing.

In 2018, Stonewall released a report[13] looking at the experiences of LGBT+ people in healthcare. It shows us that an eighth (13%) of people have experienced some form of unequal treatment from healthcare staff because they are LGBT+. When looking at trans people only this figure rises to 32 per cent. Fourteen per cent of LGBT+ people avoid treatment for fear of discrimination; 62 per cent of trans people said they had experienced a lack of understanding of specific trans health needs by healthcare staff.

The most shocking is that in the UK, one in six trans people have been refused care by a healthcare service because they are trans.

When we look at these stats, we understand that even when LGBT+ people can access the services that they need there is still a disparity of how we are treated vs the cis hetero cohort.

Changing the systems, protocols and access to funding pathways might seem like an unclimbable mountain. But at the very least, once

---

13   www.stonewall.org.uk/system/files/lgbt_in_britain_health.pdf

LGBT+ people get into your service, clinic or business, having the necessary knowledge, vocabulary and ability to deliver adequate care, and understanding the differences that this LGBT+ family may have or need because of who they are or who they love, is achievable.

CHAPTER 3

Minoritized LGBT+ Folks

Be mindful that the LGBT+ community isn't exclusively white, exclusively middle class or exclusively atheist. It also isn't pie or inclusivity top trumps – a battle to justify who is the most deserving of support, love or inclusion. There is enough inclusivity, love and support to go around if we make the choice to do so.

As a doula, I spend a lot of my time going over facts and figures with clients, so that they can make their own informed decision about their care.

As an out and proud doula, when LGBT+ people come to me in need of support there isn't one single study that focuses, specifically, on the birthing outcomes of LGBT+ parents (how happy people were with their experiences, as well as their physical outcomes, rates of birth by caesarean section, induction of labour, maternal and infant mortality).

There is limited research into the birth outcomes of black and brown people, although the MBRRACE study[1] shows us that while white women die at the rate of eight in every 100,000, 15 out of every 100,000 Asian women die – over twice as many as white women – and black women have five times the risk, with a shocking 40 out of 100,000. This is in the UK, not globally.

The immediate reaction from most is to blame black bodies. That they are somehow less able to birth, or there are socio-economic

---

1   www.npeu.ox.ac.uk/assets/downloads/mbrrace-uk/reports/perinatal-report-2020-twins/MBRRACE-UK_Twin_Pregnancies_Confidential_Enquiry.pdf

factors, that black women don't educate themselves, or can't afford to attend clinics and so on. Indeed, even Ina May Gaskin, held up as the modern mother of midwifery and a staple of the reading lists of many doula and midwifery courses, said herself that if black women got into their gardens and prayed more, they might die less in childbirth and the child bearing year.[2]

However, on the African continent and in the Caribbean, when you remove the socio-economic issue, they are not at more risk than white women, so the black and brown people birthing in the country they were born and raised in have similar outcomes to white women. When they are born and raised in the UK, that is where the disparity starts. So, it is the microaggressions and the systemic and structural racism that they live and birth within that can put them at increased risk.[3]

So, what does this mean for those who fall into both groups?

We already know that LGBT+ individuals are more likely to struggle to get the help that they need from healthcare providers and that many healthcare professionals feel that they lack the understanding, experience and training to support or offer their services inclusively.

We already know that LGBT+ folk, especially trans people, are at increased risk of suicide, unemployment, homelessness and certain cancers and other health conditions, with trans women of colour being the most at risk of physical and emotional abuse and murder.[4]

There are many people leading the way in trying to unpick the reasons and find solutions to improve the system that causes the disparities for people of colour who birth, in particular Mars Lord from Abuela Doulas.[5]

It is necessary for you all to read further about the disparities that black and brown families experience when they birth their babies, and in the days, weeks and months following, as even in 2020 black

2   https://rewirenewsgroup.com/article/2017/04/26/ina-may-gaskin-racial-gaffe-heard-round-midwifery-world
3   www.npeu.ox.ac.uk/mbrrace-uk
4   www.ncbi.nlm.nih.gov/pmc/articles/PMC4205968
5   https://abueladoulas.co.uk

babies had a 45 per cent increased risk of neonatal death compared to white babies.[6]

Robert Mugabe famously said that homosexuality is 'un-African' and a 'white disease', but according to Bernadine Evaristo, 'Homosexuality existed in Africa long before the colonisers. "It's homophobia, not homosexuality, that was imported to Africa."'[7]

In the gypsy and traveller community, we also see a disparity in access and uptake of healthcare services. Despite pockets of good practice, it is known that many gypsies and travellers still find it difficult to access health services.[8] Lack of access is not simply an issue pertaining to nomadism, it also applies to sedentary gypsies and travellers. It is caused in part by a complex relationship of multiple issues to do with discrimination, marginalization, lack of trust and low expectations on the part of other agencies. Both gypsies and travellers who are 'highly mobile' and those who are settled experience difficulties, but these vary with accommodation status. Those who are highly mobile due to frequent evictions from sites experience high levels of uncertainty and anxiety caused by displacement and, sometimes, separation from their extended family groups. Settled travellers can experience high levels of depression linked to loss of their traditional lifestyle. Both groups experience discrimination.[9]

We also see disparity in the risks for those who birth while fat or plus size.[10] I am a card-carrying member of the fat positivity club (but note, not 'body positivity', as this has been hijacked by slightly chubby, at a push femme, AFAB people who make t-shirts with Body Positive slogans on, but only up to a size 14). We see fat parents refused water births, told they cannot have home births and that they must have additional scans. I used to joke that unless the cheesecake I was eating

---

6   www.ndph.ox.ac.uk/news/report-on-baby-deaths-in-the-uk-highlights-increased-risk-for-bame-and-deprived-women

7   www.theguardian.com/commentisfree/2014/mar/08/african-homosexuality-colonial-import-myth

8   www.gypsy-traveller.org/wp-content/uploads/health-brief.pdf

9   www.gypsy-traveller.org/wp-content/uploads/health-brief.pdf

10 https://assets.publishing.service.gov.uk/government/uploads/system/uploads/attachment_data/file/844210/Health_of_women_before_and_during_pregnancy_2019.pdf

was transferring into the fat only inside my vagina I thought I would be okay. Since those days, I have come to realize that it is further systematic oppression of women and those assigned female at birth. The patriarchy tells us that women and those assigned female at birth are hysterical, and in addition that fat women are lazy, uneducated, would rather be at home eating the aforementioned cheesecake than going to antenatal classes.

I was 'refused' a water birth for my first child, Isabel now eight (and a half, they will hasten to add), because they would need to get a winch to lift me if they needed to get me out quickly in an emergency. When the midwife asked how would I get out of the pool in an emergency during the home water birth I was planning if my husband couldn't lift me, my husband shrugged and said he would cut it. 'But water will go everywhere,' she insisted. 'Yes, but it's a life-or-death emergency as you are saying, such an emergency that we couldn't wait a few moments for AJ to get themselves out with some assistance for me, the doula and the midwives in attendance? It's a blow-up pool. I'll cut the thing, fuck the water!' This is clearly not a possibility in a hospital setting with those lovely huge bath-type birthing pools, but in our situation, it was viable to cut the pool, although not something that was on the midwife's radar.

So, by understanding that those at this intersection of multiple risk need more support than ever, we further cement that respecting people's pronouns, making space and the inclusion of LGBT+ people aren't just polite added extras, but could be lifesaving.

CHAPTER 4

LGBT+ and Neurodiversity

It took me a while to decide whether to include a chapter on neurodiversity and the link that is emerging with LGBT+. As a parent to an autistic child, who will one day be an autistic adult who may birth their own babies, I want to discuss the issue. I don't want neurodiversity to be blamed as the 'cause' of a person's LGBT-ness, or indeed the other way around.

Autism ruled our lives for a few years while going through the battle of diagnosis with the NHS, and eventually we gave up entirely and paid to go private at The Portland in London – a very privileged option to have had. My eldest is nearing nine now, and apart from a few areas, we can exist largely unobstructed by this world which is geared for neurotypical people.

The words that follow are written by doula and Maternity Voices Partnership (MVP) chair Nicki Burnett. Nicki lives in Cornwall, England. She identifies as a cis, bisexual, autistic woman.

I first met Nicki on Facebook parenting groups where we bonded over the breast-/chest-feeding advice she gave me with my second child. She was invaluable to our success. We chatted more as I started my doula training, and when gender diversity was attacked in a large doula organization, she stood next to me, listened to me for hours on the phone, held space for me to speak, and answered the emails when I was too exhausted with the emotional labour of it all.

When I wanted to broach this subject, I knew exactly who to go to.

Autistic birth experiences

Birth can be an overwhelming time. The raw emotion, the physical sensations, the psychological hardship, the new relationships. There are huge changes happening within the body as well as outside the body. Pregnancy and birth can take its toll on all people who experience it, but when you are experiencing it as someone who is neurodiverse in a system that is made to cater to neurotypical people, it can be almost impossible.[1,2] Autistic women experience greater difficulty with communication, anxiety and over-stimulation in healthcare settings than neurotypical women and this becomes more difficult during pregnancy and childbirth.

The way neurodiverse people see and experience the world around them is unique; we are often seen as 'too sensitive' or 'over dramatic'. We experience sensations within our own bodies differently too. We may have difficulty communicating what we are feeling, and this can be extremely important during pregnancy and birth.

Every autistic person is different, and their experiences are different. Some may be highly sensitive to pain, and health anxiety can be very real, which can lead to lots of stress and worry and feelings that there are lots of medical complications with the pregnancy that may not be medically accurate. This person will need lots of reassurance and information to allow them to understand and have realistic expectations of symptoms. However, some autistic people have been shown to have an extremely high tolerance for pain and struggle with being able to communicate what they are physically feeling. Their symptom reporting may be significantly affected. While their pain threshold may be high,

1   Lum, M., Garnett, M. and O'Connor, E. (2014) 'Health communication: A pilot study comparing perceptions of women with and without high functioning autism spectrum disorder.' *Research in Autism Spectrum Disorders, 8*(12), pp. 1713–1721. https://eprints.qut.edu.au/79943/1/79943.pdf

2   Suplee, P., Gardner, M., Bloch, J. and Lecks, K. (2014) 'Childbearing Experiences of Women With Asperger Syndrome.' *Journal of Obstetric, Gynecologic & Neonatal Nursing, 43*(1), p. 76, doi: 10.1111/1552-6909.12455

their sensitivity to touch, and sensory input, may be significantly reduced.

This can have an impact during labour, especially in a hospital environment. My experience with my first child highlights this. I found during my labour that while I coped well with the pain, to the extent that nobody believed I was in labour right up until I was 10cm dilated, I struggled a lot with lights, touch, sounds and smells. Having my blood pressure taken was torture and the very few vaginal examinations I had were truly horrific. I didn't understand what was happening, I was woefully unprepared and had lots of medical professionals ignoring my feeble attempts to communicate. My sensory capacity was absolutely taken over by the sensations of labour and birth, and being touched without warning or consent was incredibly difficult for me. I'm sure the midwives thought they were being helpful by touching me and stroking me, but I couldn't vocalize how much I hated it. The overwhelming stimulation caused me to completely shut down and become non-verbal. I couldn't hold a conversation until hours after my son was born.

Symptom reporting can be highly affected. When not pregnant, I have trouble with understanding the feelings within my body. This is called interception and can range from knowing when I am hungry or thirsty, recognizing when I need to use the toilet to being able to understand where pain is coming from and explain how it feels. It can also affect temperature control. During pregnancy, this can be even more of an issue, as while we try to understand the changes happening within our bodies, everything feels different, our internal organs are being moved around our body cavity and then we have a growing human being kicking us in the ribs and punching our bladder. This can be very stressful and tiring, we can become dehydrated easily especially in hot weather and can miss symptoms of early labour as well as early signs of complications. We may struggle to recognize changes within our own bodies or may report them differently. It is important that our caregiver really listens and can ask the right questions to ensure important changes are not missed.

The way autistic people communicate can be quite different from neurotypicals, especially in times of high stress or overwhelm. We can often be called aggressive when really we are trying to communicate our feelings while dealing with our body's reaction to stimulus. Seeing multiple different people during pregnancy and labour means that we do not get time to build a relationship or trust with anyone, the people trying to communicate with us probably won't understand our needs and will often misinterpret what we are trying to say.

Communication during appointments can also be affected by the environment we are in. Most appointments are held in hospitals or doctors' surgeries, and these environments can be difficult for neurodiverse people. The lights, smells and sounds can take a lot of processing and lead to a person feeling overwhelmed just by sitting in the waiting room. This means that by the time we get into the appointment (often late, which is a whole different issue!), we are already beyond our capability to communicate effectively. It takes us much longer than the ten-minute allotted time to explain how we are feeling and ask what we need to ask. We end up feeling rushed, more stressed and often we either shut down or melt down, meaning we are often judged again as aggressive, uninterested or unintelligent.

Having a newborn baby is also a huge sensory experience, and the demands a baby puts on a neurodiverse person can be tough and overwhelming. The constant sound and smells, the baby's need to be held, breast-/chest-feeding can all contribute to sensory overload. Normally, after a very intense and overwhelming experience I need a good amount of alone time to recover. I need to be in a dark and quiet environment with very few demands put on me to reset. After birth, which is maybe the most intense experience in life, a neurodiverse person is then expected to instantly be a parent: to have the baby skin-to-skin straightaway, to feed the baby and often to care for the baby alone with very little support, especially if there is a stay in hospital. Ensuring enough support is in place to allow the neurodiverse person to recharge and not feel overwhelmed is important.

So, support and communication are key issues. Listening without judgement, allowing enough time to effectively communicate and enable the neurodiverse person to ask questions and process information, and trying to keep the environment as unstimulating as possible are important factors. Can you meet them at their home or in an environment where they are comfortable? Continuity and a trusting relationship can make a huge difference to a neurodiverse person during childbirth, as everyone reacts differently. It's important to get to know a person's triggers and how they communicate so that the appropriate support can be provided during labour.

Not all LGBT+ people are autistic, but 7.8 per cent of adolescents with gender dysphoria are autistic, whereas in the general population autistic people represent 1 per cent.[3]

---

3   https://www.ncbi.nlm.nih.gov/pmc/articles/PMC2904453

CHAPTER 5

How Did You Even Get Pregnant Anyway?

There are many ways that people may choose to start a family. Even in cis hetero circles, it isn't always achieved by the 'old-fashioned' way. Sperm and egg donation is a complex system with laws and procedures, and other barriers such as funding and availability are, like some other NHS services, a postcode lottery.

There are legal implications, and it is possible that anyone you are supporting will have sought legal advice in their decision-making process and journey so far.

The main barriers are known and unknown donors. This is self-explanatory in that known means you know the donor; they may be a friend or someone who sells their sperm privately. Unknown can be a private arrangement but usually this refers to someone who has donated to a licensed clinic and is, in the UK, unknown apart from some basic information such as their country and year of birth, height, eye colour.

Although the term is often used for comic relief, I think we would all be surprised at the number of 'turkey baster' babies and adults now in our world. This route may be taken if someone wants to use a known donor, and if they went to a clinic, they would not be able to use their chosen donation with signing away rights. The choice is sometimes about cost, waiting lists, red tape and the like. Additionally, some families feel that they have no choice but to go down this route to avoid the risk of being discriminated against by a healthcare professional.

The implications for legal parenthood are complex. The basic rule is that two AFAB people who are in a civil partnership or married at the time of conception will both automatically be recorded as parents of the child. So too for those couples not married or in a civil partnership when using a licensed clinic, but those who are not civil partnered or married when they conceive their babies at home or by private arrangement leaves the non-birthing parent having to adopt the child to obtain parental rights and parentship.

LGBT+ individuals and cis/straight people alike use at-home insemination as well as fertility clinics. Some further examples are detailed briefly below.

Egg donation: By its nature this is carried out in a clinic. This may be two AMAB people or two or more people whose own eggs are not viable for insemination.

Co-parenting: Two (or more) people who may or may not have the biology between themselves to make a baby but are not in a relationship. A gay man and a bisexual woman, for example.

Surrogacy: There are two routes for this. 'Straight' (snort) surrogacy involves the surrogate (pregnant person) using their own eggs, and the baby is conceived at home or in a clinic. Gestational/host surrogacy means that the embryo is implanted into a surrogate. This could be the egg and sperm of the intended parents or, where not possible, a donor egg and/or sperm may be used. Currently, dual donor (where both the sperm and egg have been donated) is not legal in the UK.

In both instances there are clinics, processes and legal implications. As previously mentioned, whoever births the baby is recorded as the mother, even if they are not genetically related to the baby, so adoption or a parental order will be the next step for legal parenthood for the parents of the surrogate baby.

Adoption and fostering: Research has shown that from April 2018 to March 2019 14 per cent of all families adopting in England were same-sex couples.[1]

Since the start of adoption in the UK, single people could adopt, but until 2005 (England and Wales; 2006 for our Scottish friends[2]) LGBT+ couples could not. In Northern Ireland, although the laws changed in 2013, very few same-sex couples, a handful in fact, have been successful with this.[3]

Pregnancy isn't always straightforward. For each person there can be a multitude of reasons as to why they cannot conceive without assistance or medical intervention. First, you need to ask yourself, is there a reason you need to know this about them? You may be a midwife who needs to know the other half of the baby's DNA to ensure that you can rule out any genetic conditions or refer on to other services if needs be. If you are asking to satisfy your curiosity because its unusual and you want to educate yourself then take a step back. Remember that they are not there to educate you, no one owes you an education on their 'unusual' circumstance. If you need to ask, then deploy your questions in a sensitive manner.

With the improvements in in vitro fertilization (IVF), we are lucky to be living in a time where more people than ever can carry and birth their babies. There are also the options of surrogacy, sperm and egg donors, adoption and fostering. Some of these options are only recently available to LGBT+ folks. It is also growing in popularity; the Office for National Statistics released a study in 2013 showing us that in 2011 there were 8000 same-sex families, rising from 4000 in 2010.[4]

The following is written by Nathan Welch – he/him. Nathan is a home-birthing dad to two little people with lots of breastfeeding and milk-sharing experience. Nathan is a trans man who is on testosterone

---

1   www.cvaa.org.uk/news/10-facts-lgbt-adoption-fostering-week

2   www.stonewall.org.uk/our-work/campaigns/2002-same-sex-couples-free-adopt-adoption-and-children-act

3   www.pinknews.co.uk/2018/12/15/northern-ireland-same-sex-adoption

4   www.ons.gov.uk/peoplepopulationandcommunity/birthsdeathsandmarriages/families/bulletins/familiesandhouseholds/2018

and is married to his husband. He is also a practising full-time NHS community midwife.

I met Nathan at the Procreate Project at King's College London in 2019. A firm friendship blossomed over shared experiences as trans parents working in the birth world. Hearing Nathan talk at events as well as the incredible YouTube videos he offers on his channel 'Trans Midwife 18', I knew we had to hear from him in this book.

Trans masculine and non-binary folk who can carry, birth and feed little humans – the medical lens

Something very poorly understood is childbearing after medical transition has already commenced. Unfortunately, there is next to no research available but there are a few key things from anecdotal evidence that I can share.

Disclaimer: someone identifying as male or non-binary and using he/him or they/them pronouns is common before or without any medical intervention and their identity is valid and should be respected regardless of their outer appearance. You do not need to ever have or want any medical treatment to be trans.

Medical transition for people with reproductive organs capable of childbearing, usually with the goal to masculinize or appear more androgynous, can include the following: taking testosterone, having 'top surgery' or a mastectomy to remove breast tissue and make the chest appear masculine, and 'bottom or lower surgery', which is complex and can take several years to complete.

Testosterone: trans people who have been on testosterone for years and have grown full facial hair and appear outwardly male are able to come off testosterone, allow their menstrual cycles to return and conceive, carry and birth a healthy baby. And they have, many times.

Testosterone has several effects on the genitals of an assigned female at birth (AFAB) person; it can cause the clitoris to grow and appear and act more like a small penis. It may also cause atrophy of the vaginal soft tissues which means they can be thinner, sore, more sensitive and tear and bleed easily. This effect tends to get gradually worse the longer a person has been on testosterone. However, vaginal atrophy tends to reverse quickly after discontinuation of testosterone therapy due to oestrogen and progesterone returning to normal levels, so come the time of birth, this should cause no issues.

It is VERY important that they are no longer taking testosterone while pregnant if they want to continue with the pregnancy. Accidental conception can happen on testosterone, which is teratogenic (harmful to the foetus). When testosterone is discontinued, it is simply stopped with no weaning off period or gradual decrease and this is not harmful to the person. The healthcare professional should give this advice without hesitation:

- Immediately discontinue testosterone
- See a gender specialist doctor urgently.

BIRTH AND CAESAREAN SECTION CONSIDERATIONS
It is vitally important as the healthcare professional for a trans person that you do not make assumptions about the mode or place of birth that the person may choose. Do not assume you know what will cause a trans person's dysphoria.

Trans people often elect for home birth and midwifery unit birth with as few interventions and people around as possible, to maintain a safe space in which they are least likely to be misgendered.

However, being trans masculine or non-binary with the potential dysphoria and complex feelings about the body and childbirth is reason enough to require informed choice about elective caesarean section. If this is what the person is requesting it is important to recognize this as a valid reason for referral to consent for an elective caesarean section.

It is rarer but still possible that a trans person may have had gender confirmation surgery on their genitals before choosing to carry a child. In these circumstances, a referral to a consultant is necessary to discuss the options but it is likely that an elective caesarean section will need to be seriously considered. They may still be able to birth through their genitals but there might be a risk that surgery results will be permanently altered. This type of surgery is recognized as necessary and is accessible through the NHS – it is not to be considered as either female genital mutilation (FGM) or cosmetic surgery.

INFANT FEEDING

Trans people may be pre- or post-top surgery when they decide to carry a child. If they're pre-top surgery they may or may not plan to breastfeed/chest-feed like any other new parent; however, extra sensitivity is required here.

Some trans people prefer to refer to their breasts/chest as any number of nicknames; if in doubt, ask. For example, 'How would you like me to refer to your chest when discussing infant feeding?'

Pregnancy may affect the results of top surgery; usually during surgery (unless they have had a reduction or reconstruction) all the mammary tissue is removed so the breasts will not grow back, although natural pregnancy weight gain and the lack of testosterone might make their chest appear puffy or larger, which might feel upsetting. There can also be varying small amounts of lactation which the person may choose to use, or suppress, like anyone else.

Testosterone as a medication has a short half-life in the body of less than two weeks, so there is no concern about their human milk for their baby if they have taken testosterone in the past.

There is currently no evidence that allows us to properly assess the risks and benefits of continuing to feed their baby when re-commencing testosterone after birth, but it is likely there would be only traces in the milk and it is reasonable to assume that the benefits of human milk will still outweigh any risk of harm.

REFERRALS

Trans people may not want their gender identity clinic to know they are pregnant if they are waiting for referrals for surgery to go through – you must discuss with the individual whether they want to inform their clinic themselves or if you want to contact them.

Being trans and/or having been on testosterone and/or had top surgery in the past are not reasons to refer for consultant-led care. The only reasons to refer to a consultant are:

- having been on testosterone during the start/some of the pregnancy
- where caesarean section is being considered for any of the above reasons.

Trans AFAB people who have not had a hysterectomy should be offered smear tests.

*

Important topics of conversation are raised in this piece from Nathan. Normally, the first few questions from people I discuss these topics with are 'So there are no set terms then? Everyone is different? How are we meant to accommodate that?' My, usually infuriating, answer is that, yes, every single person regardless of their LGBT+ 'status' is different, and needs different care, different love, different medical interventions, or none, because that's what caring for individuals means. There is no one size fits all in birth work. Not every straight and cis person needs or wants the same care, so why would we expect LGBT+ people to? Building on the final point from Nathan, smear tests can be a sensitive subject for all who should be offered them. It is important to consider, as Nathan says, that women, AFAB people and those with uteri and cervices should be offered a smear test. In addition, those with breast tissue should be offered breast screening. The language in these documents can be dysphoric for those who need smears and are not women.

If a trans man is registered as a man in the NHS system they will miss out on being invited to these appointments, but registering as female has its own issues, in that letters may be addressed to Ms, Mrs or Miss prefixes by default, triggering dysphoria and making it more difficult to engage with these services.

The NHS is making steps to make these and other sex-specific services more inclusive with their language and systems. It recommends that health professionals should be aware that not everyone requesting or attending these appointments are women. This is the first step and many of us will be watching closely for how the NHS makes these products and services more accessible to trans and non-binary people who want or need them.

Accidental pregnancy/unwanted pregnancy

It is not guaranteed that taking testosterone alone will be incompatible with pregnancy, therefore accidental pregnancy and unwanted pregnancy are a topic that need to be considered.

Trans and non-binary folks assigned female at birth, even if on testosterone, can fall pregnant. As we know that trans and non-binary people may put off going to the doctor and may not be able to safely access the care that any other person wishing to avoid pregnancy is able to, it's not surprising that accidental pregnancies occur.

This is another reason why services catering to people assigned female at birth need to be made accessible to those who aren't women. We know that the language that is used on invitations to smear tests disengages the trans and non-binary community and leads to them putting off these tests (if they would have had them otherwise – some people choose not to have them at all and that is their choice).

Women's clinics are often filled with heavily gendered language, even before setting foot in the system. Ringing up with a deep voice asking for an appointment to a women's clinic could be met with confusion and a refusal to grant the appointment unless the woman herself calls to ask for the appointment.

It is also possible that a trans or non-binary person will have an unwanted pregnancy through rape. The 2015 U.S. Transgender Survey found that 47 per cent of trans people are sexually assaulted in their lifetimes.[5] The highest rates are, unsurprisingly, among black and brown trans and non-binary folk.

Rates increase as the lack of supportive family and loved ones increases the risk of homelessness, which increases the risk of job insecurity, which increases the risk of incarceration, and so on.

Better access to clinics and healthcare professionals for treatment and counselling in these circumstances is sorely needed.

Reproductive rights

A widely accepted definition of reproductive health is 'A state of physical, mental, and social wellbeing in all matters relating to the reproductive system. It addresses the reproductive processes, functions, and system at all stages of life and implies that people are able to have a satisfying and safe sex life, and that they have the capability to reproduce and the freedom to decide if, when, and how often to do so.'[6]

The World Health Organization (WHO) defines sexual health as a state of physical, emotional, mental and social wellbeing in relation to sexuality.[7] It is not just the absence of disease, dysfunction or infirmity. Sexual health requires a positive and respectful approach to sexuality and sexual relationships, as well as the possibility of having pleasurable and safe sexual experiences, free of coercion, discrimination and violence.

For sexual health to be attained and maintained, the sexual rights of all individuals must be respected, protected and fulfilled.

Most adults are sexually active, and good sexual health matters to individuals and communities. Sexual health needs vary according to factors such as age, gender, sexual orientation and ethnicity. However, there are certain core needs common to everyone, including high-quality information and education, enabling people to make

---

5   https://transequality.org/sites/default/files/docs/usts/USTS-Executive-Summary-Dec17.pdf
6   www.who.int/westernpacific/health-topics/reproductive-health
7   www.who.int/reproductivehealth/publications/sexual_health/defining_sexual_health.pdf

informed responsible decisions, and access to high-quality services, treatment and interventions.

Access to NHS treatment

There are currently no hard and fast rules or availability on egg or sperm freezing before medical transition. There is no guarantee that the NHS will help anyone needing these services. It is very much still a postcode lottery. It is essential for each person to speak to their local authority as the clinical commissioning group (CCG) in their area holds the funds for these services.

This may understandably be a deciding factor in whether people start medical transition if they know that they may not be able to guarantee their ability to conceive or store their sperm or eggs for a later date.

It would be an act of allyship for you to know what the process is and what funding is available in your area for trans people who may want to store their gametes.

Of course, there are families that conceive their babies without any assistance. One family I have supported as a birth and postnatal doula in East London did just that.

An interview with Rivers and Martha

Rivers and Martha came to me in the summer of 2019. They were both keen to have a doula who not only was queer competent but themselves had lived experience of existing in a world as a trans person.

Rivers was pregnant with their second child. They told me, over a ludicrously expensive coffee on the South Bank, that as their identities intersect at so many points of disparities – black, disabled, trans as well as being an American with limited experience in the systems and processes of the NHS – they really wanted someone to walk with them during this journey. They wanted someone who could, if needed, provide some comfort, reassurance and love. Rivers and Martha also had a further juncture with their intersectionality. Martha is a trans woman. Within a few minutes of meeting Rivers, I had that feeling that doulas and other birth workers reading this will know all too well. That feeling of falling in love with your clients or service users. Their funny, assured and warm nature immediately fitted with mine and I was overjoyed when they asked me to be their doula a few days after our meeting.

I spoke to them as C, their baby, was reaching 15 months old. I hadn't seen them in nearly a year as the pandemic had made it impossible for us to meet in person. It was so wonderful to see them again, and my, C had grown!

It is so necessary to hear the stories of families like Rivers and Martha. Their story, similar to my own, of LGBT+ families who have the biology themselves to make a baby are often overlooked. Not all LGBT+ families will need fertility treatment. The entirety of LGBT+ competency cannot focus on pathways for funding for sperm donation, or adoption regulations. It goes deeper than that. Rivers can tell us what it is like to move through these cis heteronormative insisting systems as a pregnant, black, disabled, non-binary person. Martha can give her voice to trans women who are mothers – whose voices are so often simultaneously silenced and beaten back, and hardly ever heard.

Martha: 'I am lucky enough to have my gametes stored on the NHS. It took a long time to get it sorted; the funding and the logistics and so on all took ages. The whole time I had to be off HRT, which was frustrating. When we then decided we wanted a baby, because we have our eldest child, F, who is six now, they wouldn't give us funding.

Rivers: The fact that we already had a baby meant they wouldn't fund another one, so to speak. Even though the gametes are already stored, and being paid for continuously, we had to pay to be inseminated.

Martha: I don't have a legal connection to F but because Martha does, that was enough for them to be able to deny the funding.

AJ: So, because one of you had a baby, together you wouldn't get funding?

Martha: Yeah, basically. They still have my gametes in storage, but would have to wait until we can pay about £5000 per pop.

Rivers: Nice! Don't say pop, haha!

AJ: £5000!

Martha: Yeah, £5000 with no guarantees at the end of it. It could take one attempt, it could take several attempts to conceive.

AJ: So, the NHS would pay for the storage, and they still are paying for the storage of your gametes, but you still have to pay to access them.

Martha: Yes, but I did get in right at the end (of when they were funding freezing for storage of gametes). The NHS doesn't typically pay for that now. It was a really convoluted process that took about two years. The whole time I was off HRT. Most trans people are told that if they start HRT that it may make them infertile. If a trans person hasn't had any bottom surgeries, then there is no proof that HRT will make you infertile. So having to be off HRT for so long while waiting for these tests, clearances, funding requests to go through can be really damaging. It is hard to get a doctor to tell you that though.

AJ: That is a common thing I have been told by most trans people who have taken HRT. They have been warned and told at most appointments and junctures that this will or could make them infertile.

Martha: Sometimes you have to ask the question without the trans element to it. I might ask what if a cis man was taking HRT and then came off it, or an AFAB person was taking HRT, would that be okay? Usually, they know the answer to that, but when you add this layer of trans-ness then answers become less available to them, for some reason!

AJ: We had this after C was born, didn't we? We were asking about medications and breast-/chest-feeding and we were really struggling to find an answer relating to a trans woman.

Martha: Yeah, but then if you look for the answer for cis people you are more likely to get it.

Rivers: Given that we couldn't use the stored gametes, Martha had to come off HRT, again. We had to wait a period for the HRT to get out of her system.

Martha: Yes, about four or five months.

Rivers: We did the 'usual', erm, 'baby dance' route. I don't know if that is too much information!

AJ: I do think that it is so underrepresented. So many people think that if you are talking about LGBT+ conception that you will be dealing with donors or surrogates and that isn't always the case.

Martha: I think it is something that is more common than we think. Most of the trans women I know have made their babies in the 'traditional' way. Even if like me, it was after they had transitioned.

Rivers: Additionally, we did try at-home insemination. We wanted to stack the numbers in our favour.

Martha: I took some incredibly gendered vitamins: Men Vitamins, Go Faster Striped Vitamins, Manly Man Vitamins. It was so ludicrous at times it went beyond funny and into sad.

Rivers: I was tracking all my cycles and everything like that, and in the end, I think it took about four months or so.

Martha: I went off hormones long before that though, so if you count that time, it goes on for about a year.

Rivers: There we are, it isn't the most romantic conception story, haha!

AJ: They seldom are though; I think that is just a rose-tinted view of the world though!

Rivers: We have also thought about if we want more children. The pregnancy for me was difficult and I don't know if I want to do that again. Now Martha is back on HRT it seems like too much to battle against.

Martha: For me anyway, personally. Having been on HRT and seen what my body can do, I have that experience now of being on HRT and seeing my body further align with who I am. I wouldn't mind having to come off again if that is what we had to do to get another beautiful baby. But, for some people that just wouldn't be an option.

Rivers: It is so frustrating that we have gametes sitting there that we cannot use.

Martha: We asked if we could just have them, to try at-home insemination, but they wouldn't let us!

AJ: I am guessing they must send them to a registered clinic or something?

Martha: Exactly that, yes. They can send them to another centre. You can pay £1100 for a syringe attempt but that doesn't have as high a success rate as other options, so it didn't seem worth it. Or they can destroy them, but you can't get them without paying thousands of pounds.

AJ: When you say that the pregnancy was difficult, Rivers, do you mean physically or emotionally? Was that down to 'regular' pregnancy stuff or was it trans related too?

Rivers: I think that being non-binary and pregnant had something to do with it of course but also just physically, it's a big toll on anyone. Especially then with the chest-feeding on top. It felt like something you can do in service of something that you really want; it's not a bad trade in the end for our beautiful C, but it was hard.

AJ: I think that is another really important point. So many people think that all trans people hate their pregnancy bodies. As much as some cis people enjoy their pregnancy bodies and they have never felt more comfortable in their skin and loving it, trans people can feel that way too. There are of course some people who feel dysphoric about their bodies and the changes that happen to them, cis or trans. It's like this means to an end for some people. I don't love it, but I don't hate it, it's just what my body must do to grow my baby, or feed my baby.

Rivers: Absolutely, yes!

AJ: So that's how we got here. Tell me about your experiences of maternity care, or perinatal care. Were there any experiences that were amazing and really affirming, or any that were not so much? I know when I was with you guys post-caesarean there was an awful lot of 'Mum, mum, mum, mum'.

Rivers: To be honest, it was all bad. As soon as you go into any of these clinics or hospitals you are just called mum, at every turn. I did feel really silenced. I'd go in already with that fear from past experiences. Even if I was ready and able to advocate for myself I had to start at the ground floor and undo those assumptions. It is just so much work. It was too much for us to do. I was already going through this huge experience of being pregnant, so much information being thrown at me and then I'd have to try to remember to say, 'Well, you've already said 50 things that are wrong or hurtful to me.' I just didn't have the capacity to do that.

Towards the end of my pregnancy, it wore us down so much that I became avoidant of going to my appointments. I know I had more appointments than usual because of my disability and my diabetes, pre-existing not gestational. By the time it came to those last few months or weeks I was just so worn out I didn't have any energy left to fight. I also found that they didn't take my different pains and stuff seriously. I know that isn't unique to me, but it just felt very dismissive. I had bad pelvic pain from 30 weeks. I told them and they just nodded and said yes, that is a thing. They didn't honour what I was going through.

Martha: They didn't even offer pain relief or referral!

Rivers: No, they didn't. I told them sometimes it's hard enough to get off the sofa and go to the bathroom. So, I asked if there was anything they could do to help, and there was nothing basically. During the birth and leading up to it when Martha was present in the hospital or at the appointments the gender stuff was amplified. It is so frustrating at it is meant to be this euphoric moment! We are growing our family, we are welcoming a new family member, and to have everything about who we are as people and as a family disrespected and not seen is difficult.

AJ: I don't know if you remember Martha, but as they were moving Rivers into a different room after C was born, and we were trying to get everything gathered up to follow them down to the other room, the healthcare worker came in and asked where Mum was, and I gestured to Martha and said, 'She's here!' Even I was sick of it at that point, even as a third person in the room!

Martha: I do remember that. It was funny.

Rivers: Haha! I didn't see that!

AJ: I just thought, if I am frustrated by this, I have no idea how they are both feeling now.

Martha: It was irritating. I don't try to pass. Sometimes I might, if we are flying and I don't want to be questioned or frisked based on the disconnect they perceive because of how I look versus my documents. I mean my voice usually gives it away in the first instance anyway. It's very normal for me (to be misgendered). Conception, pregnancy and birth are a heightened version of it though. There is a lot of 'the father', 'the dad' and so on. We sometimes would ask 'Who?' Haha! But we just got more confused looks than before when we did that. There were some aspects I really wish they had had a provision for, like the language in conception or language on the notes, to put me down as biological parent or something like that. Additionally, if we had another baby, I am confident that I would be able to breastfeed that baby. But, only due to copious amounts of research by ourselves. Also, luck, that my GP gave me new hormones. Getting the cyclic HRT was a whole thing. My GP said she had to consult her legal team and back it up with all this evidence. Think how much your GP must like you to do all those steps, you know? I wish there was more support for parents who aren't the gestational parent but are women, or who have breasts that want to breast- or chest-feed.

AJ: Such a lack of information. Then when you add this layer of transness it is another level of difficult.

Martha: The cyclic HRT has made a huge difference to my breast tissue growth, which makes it easier for latching and stuff like that. C being here made a huge difference. I had some growth when I became a mother too. The hormones I suppose!

AJ: Absolutely!

Rivers: I did want to share a couple of good moments. In the ward I was staying in the night before my caesarean section partners weren't allowed to stay. The midwife who had been caring for us for a few hours in that ward went out of her way to get us a single room so that we could be together.

AJ: I remember you telling me about that; that is lovely.

Martha: There was also one scan where someone said parent, maybe once. They looked at me and took a pause and said 'parent' rather than father or dad, which I think would have normally been what they said in that situation. Oh, and, with C's birth certificate, I am down as parent! The person doing the appointment misgendered me and I think he was doing that to 'make it up to me' in a way.

AJ: What is the usual process for trans women then?

Martha: If we had used a clinic, I would have been able to go down as parent. Having a GRC I don't think would make a difference, because we have seen trans dads be put down as mothers when they have birthed their baby, so I assume with a huge degree of certainty that I would have gone down as father otherwise. So trans women can go down as parent if you use a clinic but father is the default if not. We didn't use a clinic, but I still got to go down as parent, so I was really pleased about that.

AJ: Are you parent 1 and parent 2 or mother and parent?

Rivers: Mother and parent.

Martha: They got it the wrong way round!

AJ: Yeah, they have flipped it!

Rivers: I feel like what it proves is that gender is not this natural reality that they pretend it to be. But it is something that they must continually and legally reinforce. So, it doesn't make sense.

AJ: Oh totally, like the Maternity Act going through the House of

Lords recently.[8] It said 'pregnant person' because that is the way it's always been written, but then you had a lot of people up in arms because the queers are removing language!

Rivers: Of course, of course!

AJ: What about after C was born? Did you have any good experiences with health visitors or baby groups and so on?

Martha: We barely tried to get people to do the 'them' thing with C. It was too much hard work. We were so tired from trying to advocate for ourselves that we had run out of steam to advocate for C.

Rivers: Yes, at that point we had just given up. I do remember that with F, our eldest, the health visitor put them in the red book as sister. I remember thinking, 'Wow, cis people are wild.' They had seen F playing across the room and had assigned them all these expectations and assumptions, based on what? I couldn't even work out what had led them to that assumption. Their name is unisex. Was it their clothing, maybe? Was it their hair? The toys they were playing with at that moment? I don't know. Weigh clinics would always be an event. We dress the children in clothes they like, or clothes that we like before they can show us a preference. C would be dressed in the markings associated with one gender, and once they were being weighed, without their nappy the staff would flip their language. It just seemed like far too much work to make these assumptions then change them. As for treatment of Martha and myself, it was the same. Just this assumption of who we are.

C also had a urinary tract infection, so we had some medical dealings in the first few weeks. I found the paediatricians to be better as they are not in this mindset of 'mum this, mum that'.

If we were to go through it all again, we talked about what we could do to make it a more affirming experience. Apart from making

---

8   www.bbc.co.uk/news/uk-politics-56204865

it this big fight at every turn, I don't know what we could do. You also don't want this experience to be a fight. It shouldn't have to be. You don't want all the appointments and milestones to be marred with this undertone of conflict.

AJ: I hear you. It's this toss-up between investing emotional energy in educating or explaining, which could potentially reveal you to a homophobe or a transphobe. Or they won't understand, and you will need to invest even more energy and time in them. It is possible they might get it, and everything will be great, with a few slip-ups but nothing too bad. But, that seems unlikely when there are so many different people you meet throughout the whole journey. I totally get why saying nothing and taking the path of least resistance is the best option for some families.

Rivers: We just felt lucky that we were in a privileged position to be able to have private aspects of our care. We couldn't go fully private to clinics where we knew they have experience of helping and caring for families like us. But we could access a queer doula, not just someone who was queer competent or affirming but someone who was queer themselves. We were able to get an International Board of Certified Lactation Consultant who helped us with our feeding journey. Would we have felt comfortable getting that support from an unknown service? I am not sure we would have done. Each time you must engage with a different or new service it's a roll of the dice if it is going to help you or if the cost of explaining yourself or being erased entirely is worth it. I would wonder if they have even thought that families like ours exist.

Martha: It's not just that people haven't thought about it though. This was proven by when I would go to appointments in jeans and a t-shirt and would get called the father, but then, if I went in heels and a dress, I would still get called the father. So even when we 'perform' ourselves the way they expect us to, it still doesn't work. I am sure that some people just need to think for a minute and remember the word parent!

But also, some people are just horrible and will go out of their way to ensure that they reinforce their cis het assumptions on you.

AJ: Yes! There is a big difference between slipping up and saying mum or dad because you are so used to saying those things to people at that time and doing so out of malice. However, some people do and will go out of their way to misgender you because they don't 'agree'.

Rivers: Right.

Martha: I think that a lot of the time people don't dislike me; as a person, they don't not like me. But I do make them uncomfortable. It hurts them to look at me. They must soothe themselves by reinforcing the cis heteronormative. Sometimes when people assume I am a cis woman, they will start off with she/her, and then when I speak, they immediately shift. It's painful to watch them do these language gymnastics sometimes. They feel as if they now must make up for misgendering me when they assumed I was a cis woman, so then they overuse masculine language. They try to validate me but get it all mixed up.

AJ: That sounds so much harder than asking, 'How do you want me to refer to you?'

Martha: That is all I ask for from doctors or anyone. Just ask.

AJ: What else do healthcare professionals need to hear to help provide better care?

Martha: 'How do you want me to refer to you?' is 90 per cent of it.

Rivers: The rest of it is learning the terms non-gestational or gestational parent. Don't make assumptions. The problem with blanket advice of 'don't make assumptions' is that assumptions are so normalized. They are built into the system; they are on the forms and the computer systems. Even when you ring up to get onto the maternity system and book yourself into that pathway for care, you are asked a million questions! Would it be so hard for one of those questions to be 'What do you want me to refer to you as!' Even with cis women, the mum language is too much.

AJ: Some people really do find it dehumanizing.

Martha: Even in this wildly gendered society, this is the most heightened experience of mentioning of gender. They really go for it sometimes. It seems as if they are going out of their way to mention gender for you, your partner and even the baby.

Rivers: I think that there were a few experiences that were okay. The people who just dealt with you as a single person. How are you feeling, how can I help you? Those experiences that were free from gender because there wasn't a need to shoehorn it into the situation. But like Martha says, sometimes people feel like they must, and, sadly, sometimes people will because it's violent.

Martha: I do remember at least one person asking what she should call me, and I said mother, and you could see on her face that she wasn't prepared for that.

AJ: This is what I say all the time to midwives. Midwives have incredible skills in language assimilation. If someone is saying fanny and boobs, they won't insist on saying vulva and breasts. They already have these incredibly honed skills and experience. It's just about opening that up to accept more terminology and therefore more people.

Martha: The reason that it needs to be clear and explained like that is because of homophobia and transphobia, regardless of whether they consider themselves homophobic or transphobic or not. If you won't switch language for a trans person but you will switch language because of a preference for a cis person, then it can't be anything else but transphobia.

An interview with Helen Green, registered midwife with Brighton and Sussex University Hospital (BSUH)

I met Helen through the general ether of the LGBT+ birth world. Helen uses they/them and she/her pronouns. They asked me to be on the panel of external reviewers for an exciting project. The project was guidance for other trusts on how to care for trans and non-binary people who are accessing maternity care. To say I was shaken was an understatement. That feeling never really went away when talking to Helen, and Ash Riddington, both midwives, and both absolute power houses in bringing trans and non-binary care out of mild whispers of hearsay to where it is, a grown-up, proper document with NHS logos on it! Helen and Ash have done incredible work here and it's so important for a few reasons.

First, this is the only document that currently exists, written by an NHS trust for other trusts to refer to or use to strive towards attaining the level of care they give at BSUH. From suggestions of language and terminology to continuity of carer, this document will be a game changer for so many healthcare professionals who want to do better by their trans and non-binary service users but don't know where to start. Please go and read the whole thing![9]

Under gender inclusion resources you will see several links to different documents. They range from pronoun stickers for maternity notes, if service users would find this useful, a gender inclusion poster for the walls of your clinics or staff areas, and a language preference sheet to put inside notes too. There is also a link for referral to gender inclusion midwives if you are in the BSUH area.

The top three links are gender inclusive language in perinatal services, perinatal care for trans and non-binary people, and support for a trans and non-binary people patient information leaflet. The leaflet

---

9   www.bsuh.nhs.uk/maternity/our-services/specialist-support/gender-inclusion

lets service users know what services are available and who the gender inclusion midwifery team are.

The gender inclusive language document starts with its mission statement as to why this is needed. It states:

> The vast majority of midwifery service users are women, and we already have language in place they are comfortable with. This is not changing, and we will continue to call them pregnant women and talk about breastfeeding. Adding to the language we use, and that people are comfortable with, ensures we are providing individual care for every person.

You would be forgiven for assuming that this was a complete wipe clean of any gendered language for all midwives at all trusts no matter who they are caring for. That is what the press reported. Several tabloid newspapers and journalists felt the need to publish misleading at best, and violent at the worst, articles with headlines that made it sound as if all language would be erased and replaced in gender natural style.

It's no surprise that the press did this. The press has a long history of creating division against all marginalized or oppressed communities, and the defaults of the world. It's not hard to see that 'Brighton Hospital tells midwives to use terms like "birthing parent" and "chest-feeding" instead of "mothers" and "breastmilk" because they risk offending transgender people' will sell more papers than 'Brighton Hospital creates sorely needed guidelines for caring for trans and non-binary parents.'

Find a headline about a trans person that doesn't use quotation marks around their gender or chosen name; doesn't italicize their gender; doesn't use 'sex change', 'she male', 'half man half woman' or similar vernacular. You'll be there a while. The violent way the press reports on LGBT+ people, more so with trans and non-binary people, isn't an accident – go and read *Trans Like Me* by C.N Lester.[10]

---

10   Lester, CN (2017) *Trans Like Me: A Journey for All of Us*. New York, NY: Virago

The quote 'In the old days men had the rack. Now they have the press' from Oscar Wilde springs to mind.

Helen and Ash were prepared, as were the others of us named on the document as external reviewers, for some press coverage but nothing like this. Radio phone-ins, TV coverage with midwives and lay folk calling in to express their sorrow and disgust that BSUH had created such a document to help us. The distain that trans and non-binary people won't just go away. That we exist. That we love. We have babies and we are already giving birth in 'your' hospitals, sitting in 'your' waiting rooms, and that maybe (definitely) because of the way the world treats us, we might require a little insulation from the sub-zero permafrost of the world's attitudes towards us.

So, after the dust had settled a bit, I was elated to have the chance to sit down with Helen – but without Ash unfortunately, as he had a prior commitment – to discuss with her directly what she wanted to tell you about this essential and joyful work.

AJ: What do you want to say to healthcare professionals who have read this book, or read the BSUH documents? What do they need to know now?

Helen: I think that the important thing is that there are two documents. The first supports the language change. It was written because there were no national guidelines and whatever we wrote would be held up as the standard or to very high standards. We always work within evidence-based care in the NHS, and it had to be robust in its research, so it wasn't just seen as a decision by a couple midwives in the trans community. We had to communicate why it was a statutory, legal and professional responsibility of midwives to use individualized language preferences, and how to implement it. The second document is how to provide clinical care in the trust: how do you do it, and how do you make a difference to those individuals? Each document serves a different purpose.

The language document is there to set the standard for what we believe would improve outcomes for trans and non-binary service users. The clinical care document is more of the practical, clinical side of stuff.

Both documents are important, and both need to be read. The approach we took for the language document is from a health inequality framework, an access framework and a human rights framework. We know that access impacts health inequalities. So, we looked at individualized approaches of care for the clinical document. We spoke to many of our service users as well as other lay people to gauge what would be most useful and impactful for trans and non-binary people moving from maternity services. The other important thing that we have to say is these are skills that healthcare professionals already have. We say this when we do any of our trainings; you arealready used to using language that service users find comforting, you are used to changing words that you might use yourself about your own body to what the service user is more comfortable with. You already have these skills. You might not necessarily have used them in this context, but you already have the necessary skills to do this and do this well. All the adjustments that we are suggesting could be useful for trans and non-binary service users are being offered to cis women. This includes appointments at home, someone to accompany you to scans, caesarean birth by parental request and so on. We have just identified that these needs and wishes may overlap with the trans and non-binary community.

AJ: That was one of the big things when I was reading the document for the first time. It isn't a 'you must', 'you should', 'you must not'. It was an offering of: we are members of this community so we have lived experience and we have spoken to other members of this community and this is what we think might be helpful to offer people.

Helen: Yeah, it is also helping people to recognize that no matter what options you may choose or decline that it isn't a marker of how trans or non-binary you are. So personally, I wouldn't need the pronoun stickers, or the language preference sheet. I wouldn't mind having my appointments at any location, that wouldn't be a problem for me. It doesn't make me less non-binary to do that. We ask if people identify as trans/non-binary for data collection, but equally, trans or non-binary service users don't have to be referred to us. It is always the service user's choice of what route of care they would like to go down. It will be updated as well to include a referral for case loading within our trust too. Case loading has been shown to improve access for marginalized groups, it makes sense to offer that to service users too if they want that. Some of the trans and non-binary service users identified the risk of multiple contacts as a risk factor for misgendering and having to 'explain' yourself continually, so it makes sense in that way too. Our goal is to upskill all our staff; however, we know that case loading can improve access for marginalized groups, so it is a good thing to have these routes open to those who want it. It is important that all staff are upskilled and can give appropriate, brilliant care to all service users.

The alternative is that you only have the LGBT+ birth workers caring for the LGBT+ service users.

AJ: A cis lesbian I spoke to, Adelaide Harris, had similar concerns about always being the one to care for LGBT+ people. Obviously, we want to care for LGBT+ folk because they are our kin, but continually being pigeonholed into who you can or should care for is problematic. It does feel tokenistic to say we aren't going to do the work to overhaul or add to the system or language, we are just going to let the other LGBT+ people handle it.

Helen: Yes, exactly. If you are pregnant, and you have continuity of carer, that's great, that is the gold standard. But, at some point you may have to enter the wider system, through emergency admittance, extra scans, reduced movements, if you opt to have an induced labour or whatever that might be, so we need to ensure this is trust wide. We need all the staff trained because the chances are, even if all these trans folk are under a special case loading or continuity of carer team, they may need additional input from the wider system.

AJ: Yes, of course.

Helen: We also identified that those moments, the emergency admittance situation for example, would be when service users are the most vulnerable.

AJ: Yes, totally!

Helen: If something bad is already happening, you are particularly vulnerable. By the nature of midwifery care, you only access something beyond that when something is going wrong.

AJ: Thank goodness you said it. The idea that continuity of carer would solve all the problems for the LGBT+ community has many holes in it, and this is one of the biggest.

Helen: Continuity of carer will minimize poor outcomes. However, you could have the best care in the world, access to all kinds of services in health, social and mental health care and still have a complete placenta previa and need a caesarean section. That would be a lifesaving operation, but you still need the anaesthetist, the scrub nurse, the theatre nurses, the midwives over there, the receptionist in the hospital and others to be aware of how to give the best care they can.

AJ: Yep.

Helen: Everyone we have offered the service to so far has taken us up on our offer. Sometimes they don't want everything that we offer. Some people have wanted someone to come with them to their scans, but they don't feel they need the language preference sheet or the pronoun stickers. Some have enjoyed coming to their appointments in house. Others have really needed the appointments, where possible, to be at home. Cis women's experience of pregnancy is never the same so we cannot expect trans and non-binary people's experience and wants and needs during pregnancy to be the same either.

AJ: Yeah, for sure! I am really starting to get the impression that this isn't rocket science and it is all skills that healthcare professionals have already. But they might need a bit of help because they don't have any personal or lived experience of caring for or being a member of this community, so this is what your documents are doing. They provide that insight and lived experience to healthcare professionals to aid them in giving the best care they can.

Helen: One of the biggest barriers has been letting people know that the service exists. One of the big reasons we went to Trans Pride here in Brighton was so that we could set up our stall and people would know that midwifery care and our midwives will be here for them, if they want or need us, particularly for communities that have a history of trauma or mistrust in healthcare professionals because of their journey and lived experience. And again for trans and non-binary folk with the misinformation about hormones that is out there. We just wanted people to know that we exist, and that we have thought of them, and we are here. To see young trans folk at Pride talking to us and knowing that they can have a baby if they want to. To let them know that this is what the care should look like for them, we aren't going to touch them without their consent, they don't have to come to the hospital for every appointment and sit in a waiting room getting funny looks. That has brought joy to trans folk and their parents too. It was so refreshing to be a part of trans joy. We did speak with people who were sterilized to be able to access the transition that they wanted, and they never got a choice; those who were lied to about testosterone (that taking hormones will make you infertile), they never had a choice. We were standing there saying we can move forward, you can expect more from your lives, you can have the care that you want and need, and it isn't about trying to contort yourselves around care pathways that already exist. You can have something that is just for you.

One of these most powerful moments was at Trans Pride. A trans man came up to me, and I think he was in his late 20s, or something like that. He just started crying. He said his family had all been wonderful, and his friends, and he had had a great life. Until he said he might want to have a baby. He said he was made to feel disgusting and broken by some of the people who had been so supportive and loving when he came out. He said it was the first time he had held a conversation with someone who made him feel that it was okay for him to want a baby. More than that, it was the first time someone had said it was normal; it was beautiful, and it was great. He said the short conversation we had changed his life.

If I never do anything else regarding trans folks and pregnancy, that will be enough.

AJ: Every birth worker who exists, who works with people at any point during the journey to conceive, grow or birth their babies, has that ability within them to be the person you were for this young man. They might need a little bit of hand holding, they might need to listen to some podcasts, they might find it useful to read some books. But they can be this person.

Helen: Yes! Exactly! We had someone who, because they had received such incredible support throughout their pregnancy, said they felt comfortable enough to go to baby groups!

AJ: Oh gosh, love a baby group! I still speak to people I met at baby group with my eldest who is going to be nine this year. Our kids have grown up together!

Helen: What a difference these groups can make for perinatal mental health as well. Having that environment of your peers and getting out of the house to be surrounded by other people who are going through a very similar time and experience to you.

AJ: It's huge! Sometimes that was the only place I had been that week because I was worried that the baby would cry in Morrisons or down the high street or even at the park that I wouldn't be able to find a seat to sit down and feed them or something like that.

Helen: We do offer antenatal education for trans and non-binary people at home if they don't want to go to groups, but the group aspect can be so important. Luckily, because it's Brighton, we have lots of people who run groups like baby yoga that are making changes to be inclusive and to be visible in their inclusion so that more trans and non-binary parents feel welcome in those spaces.

In midwifery, we talk a lot about self-efficacy, about helping people get to the point where they feel good and capable in themselves. That is what good gender inclusive midwifery can do. It can aid people's belief in themselves. You help people know they have the right to good and decent care. That carries through to the rest of their lives. People are relatively young when they have babies, and it is hoped that they will live long and happy lives. They will have more points of contact with healthcare professionals, and we want them to go on and use those skills of self-efficacy in all aspects of their life.

We can also heal old wounds and build bridges with survivors of healthcare trauma. We have had people who have really struggled to engage with the midwifery team because of their previous experience of medical trauma – to the point that they didn't want to have any care at all from any midwives or perinatal services. But through the relationship and the trust that we could build, having these options and services available and having someone with lived experience that they know they can trust with those parts of themselves, they have had a really positive experience. I hope that the next time they need to go to the doctor they won't be so hesitant and will seek medical care if they want or need it. That is a huge gain for public health. So much of midwifery is public health; if you can increase self-efficacy, if you can increase access, if you can increase trust in the system, you improve a person's experience of public health.

AJ: It's not always about getting it right so you don't offend or upset people. It could be that getting it right will save lives.

Helen: It might take a little bit of effort, like you say, reading an article, doing a training day, listening to those with lived experiences, but it can be lifesaving.

*

My thanks again to Helen and Ash, not just for contributing to the book but for the work they have done at BSUH. This work will go on to impact and improve so many lives across the country.

An interview with Gina Kinson (she/her), Surrogate UK

Some of the families who have shared their stories with me wanted to grow their families using surrogacy. I thought it only right that I speak to someone who has been a surrogate and who can tell us about it.

This conversation with Gina Kinson, a two-time surrogate and member of My Surrogacy Journey, doesn't focus specifically on LGBT+ families and surrogacy, but is her journey and her story as a surrogate.

AJ: Thank you so much for talking to me, I really appreciate you sharing your lived experience.

Gina: The more knowledge out there about surrogacy and how health-care professionals can support surrogates and the intended parents (IPs) during pregnancy and labour the better. A lot of people get it wrong, so the more we can talk about it, and normalize these kinds of journeys, the better.

AJ: Wonderful, thank you so much. One of the questions I have been asking all the people who have been kind enough to share their stories with me is, what do you want healthcare professionals to know about surrogacy?

Gina: What I would like them to know first is that the surrogate is not the mum or the parent at any time. They are not carrying their own babies. The IPs are the parents. They are the ones who need to be addressed and included. Obviously, don't ignore the surrogate, but sometimes the focus tends to be on the surrogate. It feels as if they consider her to be the mother until the parental order goes through. That isn't the case. The IPs are the parents from conception. The surrogate and the IPs are a team, all together.

During labour, yes, the surrogate is the one in labour. At the same time, the IPs are also in labour. They are also experiencing this labour. No matter who the IPs are, whether they are LGBT+ or not, this is their labour and their experience also. Surrogates want the IPs to be involved, they want them to know all the information that they do. I think it's as simple as treating the parents as parents from the moment baby is conceived.

Some of the difficulty and hesitance from some healthcare professionals comes from the fact that the surrogate is the mother by law, until that parental order goes through. However, common sense will tell you that the surrogate would not be doing this unless they were completely aware that this isn't their baby.

AJ: I understand that there is that legal barrier and that would be concerning from a litigation point of view.

Gina: There is a very simple answer to that. Ask the surrogate! As soon as they are admitted, ask their permission: 'Can we share this information?' Consent can be verbal; it doesn't have to be written down. Therefore, if the IPs can't be there at that moment, what with Covid right now, or say that it is an emergency admittance, and they are on route, but it will take them some time to get there and they are calling for updates and to check on how the surrogate and baby are doing, you then have verbal permission to speak to them about their baby. We are just stuck in this limbo regarding laws right now. Provided the healthcare professional writes in their notes that they got verbal permission then there should be no concern for litigation.

AJ: Do you think it's just a lack of experience and knowledge of the healthcare professionals caring for surrogates and IPs that gets in the way of that, as well as the laws?

Gina: Yes, I do. I also think that there are a lot of preconceptions of what this process is like and what you can and can't do. It's also about how we are exposed to surrogacy. When surrogacy is mentioned in the press it's sensationalized as an overly dramatic or rare process. Few positive surrogacy stories are shared. There are hundreds of surrogate births in the UK every year where everything goes well. If healthcare professionals had more knowledge surrounding the law and the wants and needs of surrogates, it would be better. Surrogates won't have woken up one morning and decided to do this on a whim. It most likely is a decision that has been months if not years in the making.

Surrogacy is also incredibly empowering; the surrogate gets a lot out of it too.

The relationship that surrogates and IPs build is remarkable. Because we must discuss all possibilities, we are more aware of what IPs want than perhaps some coupled parents. We must discuss what would happen if the baby was poorly, or if a caesarean was needed. Every detail is talked about, every eventuality mulled over, until everyone is clear on what could happen.

Also, know that the term 'surrogate mother' isn't really used in the surrogacy world, because they aren't the mother. The term surrogate is just fine.

AJ: Or their name, I guess?

Gina: Yes! Or their name.

AJ: It's interesting that you bring up the sensationalist nature of the reporting about surrogacy. How it's only reported when it goes wrong, or is dramatized. The LGBT+ community share that same framing. I don't want to do that here; I want to hear about the beautiful journeys. It is important. However, I want to highlight for those reading the book when it has gone wrong so that we can learn from those experiences to try and prevent another team of surrogate and IPs going through that same experience. With that in mind, would you share with us any experiences that could have gone better, or an example of how someone got it right?

Gina: I have had two very successful journeys. We had great support and a fantastic experience from the hospitals. The first journey didn't go completely flawlessly, in terms of language and terminology for me and the IPs. However, the midwives were very helpful, a little naive maybe, but we were one of the first surrogacy teams in that hospital. They helped the mother with feeding and supported her well. They even provided somewhere for her to sleep so she could stay overnight with the baby. I am not the baby's mum so I wasn't there to change nappies or feed the baby; she is the baby's mum so it is only right that she would be able to stay with her baby and do those things.

AJ: There is a cross-over with same-sex couples who have had a baby. When the non-gestational parent wants to induce lactation there is obviously a good case for that parent to be allowed to stay and have access to the baby for the purpose of bonding and inducing lactation. However, as usually this isn't something that is allowed in most trusts, this can disrupt that process and put parents on the back foot in establishing breast- or chest-feeding. The mother, gestational parent or surrogate needs to be there for their own health needs and to be cared for. The parents who are critical to the nourishment and health to the baby also need to be there. It's another reminder of how some of the steps that are needed to improve access for LGBT+ parents would benefit other parents.

Gina: Yes of course. What a lot of hospitals fall on is how many birth partners can you have in a surrogacy team. We were very lucky to be allowed to have my two birth partners, and the intended parents could be there. It was amazing and I so appreciate that. However, a lot of surrogates have found that they are only allowed one birth partner.

The surrogate needs a birth partner and the baby's parents need to be there. We often phrase it that the surrogate is themselves one person and needs their own team. But the baby is again themselves, their own person, and needs their own team. We need the hospitals to look at the policies and ask themselves at what point do they consider the baby and surrogate separate people and that they need their own teams there to care for them.

AJ: I suppose, then, anyone supporting pregnant people and families using surrogates should ask their local trusts what their policies are for birthing partners in situations of surrogacy. So when a surrogate or the IPs ask this question, they know the answer.

Gina: Yep! That would be fantastic. A lot of the policies are very old and haven't ever been updated. Once you ask the question, sometimes that is exactly what they say, and they can very quickly get 'special' permission for IPs, and the surrogate themselves can have the support team that they deserve too.

Another key thing that surrogates miss out on is postnatal care. We often get a day two or three visit. That is just to check our overall health and wellbeing at that point. The baby gets several visits. What the surrogate misses out on, because the baby isn't with them, is that frequency of checking in. Surrogates are at risk of perinatal mental health difficulties. We often hear from surrogates that they feel lost in the days after birth. It's not because they are missing the babies, it's not about that. It's because they have gone from talking to their IPs every day and having all this interaction with healthcare professionals and then as soon as baby is born, there is nothing. No one comes to see you because the baby isn't there, you don't get all the cards and well wishes. It does almost give you a sense that the floor has been pulled out from underneath you.

It would be nice if midwives were aware of that and maybe they could make a phone call at a set time. They could ring up and ask if we want to talk about the birth. When you give birth, everyone wants to come round and see the baby. The conversation usually shifts to tell me about the birth, how long was it, are you okay, what happened at this point, and surrogates miss out on this. Verbalizing your experience repeatedly can really help you process the trauma or the experience that you have just had. Surrogates miss out on that sometimes. If midwives, doulas or health visitors were aware of that perhaps they could reach out and listen to the story to aid in that emotional recovery. It might help surrogates not to feel so alone.

AJ: There is huge base of research about how talking about birth can really help in recovery, emotional and physical.

Gina: I have seen it so many times that surrogates experience this. It's not postnatal depression or the baby blues. It is just this massive shift for them that they haven't had the chance to process it.

AJ: That makes so much sense.

Gina: Generally, it's just listening and asking. That goes with everything and everyone in life, right? Asking open questions can be powerful. Just saying: How can I best provide this support? At the end of the day, none of us is the same, none of us needs the same thing. There should be fewer assumptions of what we might want or need and more questions.

AJ: That sentiment of 'just ask' has been the closing remarks of pretty much everyone I have spoken to.

Gina: It really is as simple as that, just ask.

Interview with Jake Graf, Mermaids Ambassador, actor and transgender activist and parent

I have known about Jake and Hannah Graf for a long time, first as high-profile trans people in the UK. Hannah was a captain in the British Army when she came out as trans. Jake is an actor, an ambassador for Mermaids as well as an activist for the rights of trans folk.

When I saw adverts for a documentary on Channel 4 called *Our Baby: A Modern Miracle*, featuring the journey of Hannah and Jake to have their baby using a surrogate, I was elated. To see a documentary focusing on trans people being parents felt like another huge barrier broken. I sat down to watch it the day after it first aired, trying to keep out of the comments section through fear of the transphobia that was surely to come.

There are precious few documentaries that focus on LBGT+ parents, and considering that both parents are trans I knew it would be essential viewing for all those who want to improve their competency, services and processes for parents who are in similar shoes.

The documentary shows us the journey of Hannah and Jake looking for a surrogate and conceiving their baby using IVF. We watch as they travel, with little warning during a pandemic, to Northern Ireland when their surrogate goes into labour. I watched through teary eyes as they tried to get to their baby as quickly as possible after she was born. I knew I had to speak to Jake to ask him what he wanted birth workers to know about his and Hannah's journey, and indeed, what advice he could give for other LGBT+ folks, and non-LGBT+ folks, thinking of embarking on or going through the process of using surrogacy to have their baby.

After a few rebookings due to the third national lockdown, Christmas and childcare issues, I was finally able to sit down with Jake (on Zoom, obviously!) and listen to what he had to say.

As with other interviews in this book I have tried to keep Jake's words verbatim, only editing for context and the like.

I asked Jake to start at the beginning and tell me everything.

JG: Hannah and I have learned so much through our journey, and through doing the documentary, so now I feel we are really well placed to talk about surrogacy. We only realized through starting out on the process how little information is out there.

Most of the Facebook groups or other community support hubs and so on are cis and het based but that doesn't mean there isn't useful information there that you can use.

Surrogacy is illegal in Italy, Spain and France so Ukraine has become this hub for the world to go to for surrogacy. We went to the Ukraine stand at the fertility show in Olympia and interviewed surrogates and doctors, which sadly didn't make the cut for the documentary. We learned so much from Facebook groups and meeting other parents.

For £35,000 you can go to Ukraine and basically be guaranteed a baby, no matter how long it takes. But Ukraine is totally out for LGBT+ couples. When we were at the Ukraine stand at Olympia, they were so nice when I was doing all the talking, saying, 'Yes of course, how lovely...' When I told them we were both transgender her face just froze and her whole demeanour just changed. It was clear that we weren't welcome. It was just heart breaking.

In the US, you are talking upwards of $100,000 for surrogacy. A lot of my gay friends have gone to Canada and the US but again that is because they have more, statistically speaking, disposable income, so it might not be possible for everyone to be able to do that. Even though we were lucky to have the options we did and got our baby, it still cost us upwards of £45,000.

We have been promised by politicians and so many other people for years that change is coming to the legalities for families in the UK, but nothing is even beginning to emerge here.

We did get the feeling that we were – and I think we properly were – the first trans couple to undergo the trans and surrogacy process, and that is purely because we have the financial support from our families to be able to do that. We are very, very bloody lucky.

When we talk to people about the barriers for intended parents and the legalities it's a real mix of shock and upset. That is why there needs to be updates (to the laws), but as with most things if there is a way the government can kick something into the long grass, it will. That is why we made the documentary and why we want to do more to bring these issues to light.

Everyone has an opinion about surrogacy. Some people would tell us, while standing there with their own child, 'There are so many unwanted children in the world, you should really just adopt.' Then of course there is the 'You are ripping a baby from its mother' trope. I had friends, good friends, message me and say this. I had someone message me who I've known since school saying, 'I've been thinking about it, I've seen what you are doing in the newspaper and I really think you should reconsider. You would be literally ripping a child from its mother's stomach.' I just wanted to reply WHO ASKED YOU! Everyone seems to think they can have an opinion on how other families are formed or made up. I think that because most people can't say they know someone who is trans, or most people can't say they know someone who has used surrogacy, what we found with our surrogate Laura is that when her kids told their teachers or friends, they all thought it was incredible. It is amazing what she did for us. Laura said that every single member of her close circle, her family, her friends, bar one, said that what she was doing was amazing. There needs to be more of that, more acknowledgement that it is an incredible and beautiful thing.

In the UK, you can't advertise for a surrogate, it's not even legal to ask! Some of the agencies have such tight restrictions on who can be a surrogate. There is all the usual medical stuff like body mass index (BMI), how many babies they have had, underlying conditions and so on. When we went on TV on the *Lorraine* show, we had a lot of women get in touch with us off the back of that, but the agency wiped nine of them out, just straight off the bat! Even just if their husbands had a minor criminal record ten years ago. Our surrogate, Laura, would have been ruled out by this agency because her BMI was a bit high! We have a beautiful and healthy baby with her.

AJ: What is the purpose of agencies in the UK if they can't advertise for surrogates on your behalf?

JG: In the UK, agencies can give you the opportunity to be matched, they can facilitate the sharing of information between surrogate and intended parents, like an introduction service really.

Agencies sometimes have these 'mixer' events. You go into a big room and there are surrogates and intended families all in the same room. Hannah and I balked at that, as there is no way that in a sea of 50-odd families we would have felt comfortable to navigate that space as the only trans couple, particularly as Hannah has a deeper voice and is immediately outed as soon as she speaks.

AJ: What happens once you have found a surrogate? How do you move forward?

JG: You have to agree on everything. You must think about everything! What would happen to the baby if you (intended parents) died, what would happen if there was something wrong with the baby in the womb. It was very upsetting to talk about it all. But it is so necessary. Most couples go into it thinking, yay amazing we are going to have a baby, but we had to have conversations about what happened if Millie died while inside Laura.

Then we considered that Laura is the legal mother. We could never be listed as mother and father. That's not an LGBT+ parent thing, it is the process for all intended parents. Once the parental order goes through, you are parent 1 and parent 2, never mother or father. In the grand scheme of things, and because we are quiet pragmatic people, we realized that this is the law and the way it works. I can't speak for Hannah, because she is Millie's mother, but she can never be recorded as such. There needs to be a lot of updates and changes to the system.

Millie is my genetic child, but I couldn't be on the birth certificate. Laura was married but separated at the time, so if any man could go on that certificate, it would have been him. We are so incredibly lucky to have Millie, but these are considerations that most other families having babies don't have to think about.

In the beginning we went to the London Women's Clinic, and everyone was very kind and treated us well. I was always sort of centred because Millie was mine, so to speak, then Laura next. Hannah less so because she wasn't genetically linked and there was nothing for her 'to do' in terms of treatment, tests or check-ups. When we went to scans and stuff, everyone was very pleasant. When Laura was inseminated, Hannah did feel like she was not as involved. They were talking to me about my genetic material, which egg we are going to use and so on. Then they talked to Laura about what she needed to do or be aware of. So, I understand that they were not purposefully excluding Hannah, and I know Hannah understands. They had never dealt with a couple like us before. Usually, it would be the mother and the surrogate they would be talking to and the bloke would maybe feel a bit surplus to requirements or something, but for us, obviously, that wasn't the case.

At every scan we went to, in Belfast, even though at this time same-sex marriage wasn't even legal there, we were treated very respectfully, I must say. Sometimes they would say 'the mother' and Laura would have to correct them and say, 'No, this is the mother', and gesture to Hannah, and they would quickly say, 'Oh yes, sorry.' I don't think it was ever with any malice or bigotry, it's just so ingrained in their practice. We were all allowed into all the scans, so that wasn't ever a battle.

When Millie was born, it was under very unusual circumstances, at the start of the first Coronavirus lockdown. We were told weeks in advance that we weren't going to be allowed to be in the room when Millie was born. I know Hannah really wanted to be there, but like some blokes, I had no desire to be there at all! I thought if we are in the hospital then that would be okay, but then we were told we weren't allowed to wait in the hospital, not even downstairs or anything. So, we decided we would wait in the car, in the car park. It was Covid, so we knew again it wasn't malicious, it was necessary. It wasn't any kind of a normal situation, but they still treated us with the upmost care and love. The head midwife had explained to us that we probably wouldn't be allowed in and even Laura might not be allowed a birthing partner. Millie was born at 5.30am, and Laura's birthing partner called us to tell us that Millie had been born, and to come down. We got to the hospital and it was like something out of a horror movie. Everything was dark, everything was cornered off. We couldn't even work out how to get in the hospital because so many entrances and exits were closed off. It was like something out of the film *28 Days Later*. All the receptions were closed, and we were just so anxious to get upstairs and see our baby, but there was yellow tape everywhere blocking us from getting in. We tried calling and no one was answering, then when we did get through, they were asking us 'Where is the mother?' and in the documentary you see me getting upset. I snapped, 'The mother is here, she is with me.' Obviously Hannah is the mother, but they mean the person giving birth. I was getting quite ratty because it was that first moments with our baby that we were missing. Again, I don't think it was malicious. They were run off their feet, even before you factor in Covid. There was a woman on the unit giving birth who had Covid, so, you know, they had enough on their plate. So, I can't really speak about what normally happens with surrogates and their babies, because nothing was normal during that time. When we got up there and they brought Millie in to us and they saw the love and the pure joy when we got to hold Millie for the first time, then they got it. Maybe up until then, they didn't really get it. They brought us food, they were so kind to us and treated us just like any other parents really.

The first ten days we were in Northern Ireland, I remember the midwife coming out and saying goodbye, telling us it was such a pleasure for them to be there for us; apparently, we were the talk of the ward! I suppose surrogacy is quite unusual, let alone surrogacy for trans parents! Even in the middle of this pandemic, they were so wonderful. I am sure there was someone there saying transphobic things, but we didn't hear it, we didn't see it. We had a health visitor come to the Airbnb. Her name was Pat and she was so wonderful; she didn't even turn a hair at us or our unusual situation. Very encouraging and normal.

AJ: Are there any examples of care that could have been better? Any times that you felt excluded because you are LGBT+?

JG: One of the only times we felt let down or excluded by the NHS was with the baby classes. This was our first baby, so we were nervous. We called the NHS when Laura was pregnant, and asked if we could access the antenatal classes at our local hospital. We really thought it would be beneficial to us as new, first-time parents. We called and explained that neither of us was pregnant, but we are having a baby through surrogacy. We kept getting passed around different departments and struggling really to get the information that we needed. They said if you weren't having a baby here you couldn't have the classes. I explained that our surrogate was giving birth within the NHS and obviously wouldn't be having the classes, so somewhere there must be the budget for us as parents to have these classes. Finally, when we spoke to someone else, they weren't terribly pleasant, and just said this is the policy, deal with it. Then she said, 'These classes aren't much good anyway! You don't really need them. All they really teach you is how to get a passport.'

I explained that everyone we had spoken to who had kids said we should do these classes to listen and learn and make connections with other expectant and new parents in the area. The person on the phone was very dismissive about us needing the classes. I must say it was one of the few times we did feel discriminated against. I even said on the phone, 'We're not able to have our own children! My wife is not able to give birth to our baby, and our surrogate lives in Northern Ireland and we don't want to have her travel here so late in pregnancy to give birth away from home and her family', but they just kept saying, 'No, no, no. You can't do the classes. You can't do it here.'

Maybe it's just the first time anyone had enquired who was using surrogacy; maybe a lot of people who use surrogacy go private for their antenatal preparation or whatever, but it was probably the only time we felt discriminated against, or that we were at a disadvantage to other, 'regular' parents or families. I don't think it was a trans thing, it was probably something straight and cis people would have experienced if they had called up if they were using a surrogate as well.

AJ: This book is primarily for birth workers and how they can better support LGBT+ parents. But I can't pass the opportunity to ask you, as a trans parent and as a Mermaids ambassador, what you want to tell trans people who are considering medical transition or considering having families in the future.

JG: I speak to so many young trans guys who are so desperate to get their hysterectomy and I get it; I remember feeling the same when I was younger. I just say to them, 'Guys, calm down and think about what you are doing first! The fact that I did harvest my gametes before having surgery means that I could have Millie. If you want to be a dad in the future just take some time to consider your options before surgery.' I transitioned later than most, I didn't start until I was 28, so maybe I had a bit more patience or whatever. Hannah also had the option to freeze her gametes, although funding for that is a bit of a postcode lottery. What I would say to anyone of the age or potential to be fertile and there is any chance that they may want kids in the future, then just stop and think about it.

I wouldn't have had the ability to go to the Women's Clinic in London to have my gametes harvested before transition. I was really crippled with misery over the idea of it. After six years I was able to get to a place where I was confident enough to be able to go and sit in a waiting room – well actually, I sat in the corridor because it was so awful to sit in a waiting room like that on your own as a man. I know there are a lot of people who are at that crossroads of making a decision that could, potentially, leave them in a position that Hannah is in. Hannah will always regret that. Hannah tells all the young trans girls to hang on, if you can hang on, keep it (have your gametes frozen). We would love it if Millie was a mix of us both. Millie is still perfect, of course, but we do wish she was a mix of us both.

It seems so remarkable to so many trans people that we can be happy, we can be starting a family and that's why Hannah and I do choose to be as visible as we are and share our journey. We want trans people to know that you do deserve it, and you can do this. We get thousands of messages saying, 'Your posts give me hope I can do this; I can be happy and have a family.' I really love the messages we get from parents of trans people as well. There is an idea that when you have a kid that comes out (as LGBT+) that that's it, no grandchildren, but it's just not true. We are so proud to be one of the families that is bringing that visibility and hope, not just to trans people themselves but their loved ones as well.

Maybe the healthcare professionals need to take the time to consider that this decision (to medically transition) could limit your options in later life. For the sake of 20 minutes or whatever for trans women (but is different for trans men and again depends on funding), you could retain this option later in life.

Hannah had literally thousands of messages from women, mainly actually cis women saying, 'I wasn't able to carry my baby either and you have given me hope that we can eventually have our baby too.' I got loads of messages from trans guys too saying, 'I didn't even know we could do this, how wonderful.' There is still so much misinformation out there that taking testosterone will make you infertile, which we know is not always the case. The amount of support and love we got was incredible. The number of questions was so concerning and heart breaking – there needs to be so much more visibility and knowledge for surrogacy, and we might have some future projects to help get this information out there. Anyone who is considering surrogacy, just speak to everyone who has been through it and listen to their stories and make up your own mind what is best for you and your family.

We do remain a community where some people have never, knowingly, met a trans person. Across the board there needs to be more training, more visibility. The terminology will be difficult, and the assumptions will be difficult, such as the assumption that it will be the female bodied person who will be giving birth. A lot of people asked me when we were having a baby if I would be carrying it. That wouldn't work for me, I have worked so hard to like what I see when I look in the mirror. I have worked hard for 28 years. Some trans men want to and find it so empowering and that's fab. Remember, you cannot generalize, even in minority groups where we share the same 'label' we can't all fit in the same expectations or box. Trans people are all so different, we don't even have a sexuality that binds us together. These are just my experiences and my feelings, and many, many trans people will feel differently. There is no generalization. There is no conclusion. Just listen. If we come in and say I'm the mother, I'm the father, or I will be carrying the baby, even if it's not what you expect, just be kind and open. It sounds really twee and simplistic but that is really all it is.

*

Millie woke up toward the end of the interview and I got to see her sitting on Jake's knee. She was so interested in what her dad was saying! She is an incredibly beautiful, happy and loved child.

An interview with Sabia Wade, The Black Doula

When I was speaking to Sabia, this conversation came up very early on. She told me as a non-binary woman she is asked this a lot, especially as a professional in the industry. She was kind enough to share with me why this conversation, and the assumptions around fertility, health and desire to have kids, can be so harmful.

Sabia shared with me that she has many underlying health conditions that throughout her life have taken an incredible emotional and physical toll on her body. Carrying her babies is not something that she wants to do.

Sabia: People assume because I am in this industry that I want to have babies. They ask me all the time, why isn't this what you want? In the job that you are in? I want to ask them back, 'Do you want my medical history? Do you wanna know all about me and my body? The trauma of all of that?' Especially as a black woman, I work in this industry where I know the risks of me having a baby, yet they still ask me!

I have to find the words and the story so that whoever is asking can finally say to me, or themselves, 'Okay, that's a good enough reason for you not to want to be pregnant.'

When I have the body that I have and do the work that I do and say the things that I say, people just cannot understand that I do not want to carry my own child.

In the US we have such a history around black women always being caretakers. The connection is awful, and people don't realize that this connection is sitting in the back of their minds when I say, as a black, non-binary woman, that I don't wanna do that, and for them it's just 'Huh? Why wouldn't you?'

When I had a masculine presenting partner, then people really put me in a place of 'now you can do this'.

AJ: The social filter for what you can and can't ask people is already so much lower for LGBT+ people than it is for cis and het people. Think about cis people asking about surgeries that trans people have had when we announce that we are trans. Think about the invasive and nonessential questions same-sex couples encounter when they move through the maternity services in the world – there are examples of this happening in the stories of those I have spoken to and the case studies – so it's not uncommon. in fact, the *LGBT+ In Britain* report from Stonewall tells us:

- One in four LGBT people (25%) have experienced inappropriate curiosity from healthcare staff because they are LGBT.
- A third of LGBT+ disabled people (34%) and three in ten LGBT people aged 18–24 (30%) have experienced this.
- Almost one in four LGBT people (23%) have at one time witnessed discriminatory or negative remarks against LGBT people by healthcare staff. It is of little wonder, therefore, why so many LGBT+ people aren't out to anyone about their sexual orientation when receiving medical care.
- One in five LGBT people (19%) aren't out to anyone about their sexual orientation when seeking general medical care.
- One in seven LGBT people (14%) say they've avoided treatment for fear of discrimination because they're LGBT. Almost two in five trans people (37%) and a third of non-binary people (33%) have avoided treatment for fear of discrimination because they are LGBT.
- One in four LGBT people aged 18–24 (26%) and one in five LGBT disabled people (20%) and black, Asian and minority ethnic people (19%) have avoided treatment."

---

11   www.stonewall.org.uk/system/files/lgbt_in_britain_health.pdf

The social filter of asking LGBT+ people intrusive questions that you would never ask a straight person is so well ingrained as to be acceptable. Asking gay or bisexual men who is the top and who is the bottom has been followed by many a gasp and laughter in our cultural narrative on screen or in real life. Asking bisexual people about the genitals of their current partners is next to expected. Asking trans people about their genitals even more so.

The constant questioning of our bodies, who we love, *how* we love and trying to compare it with the cis and heteronormative is exhausting and erasing.

Sabia: When you are a part of a marginalized community, there is an assumption that because you've been through shit, you can handle shit. Even more so because our communities are smaller, and we take care of each other, there is the idea that we can handle intrusive questioning of ourselves.

Of all the labels that I carry, the most obvious of them is being black. I see assumptions of me, made about me, that wouldn't be made of others. There is this big expectation of me to be the strong one you know. I carry these assumptions because I am black, I am queer, and these identities are seen as strong, and resilient. You must be the strong one out of your community – the strong black woman who can handle everything!

AJ: Have your experiences shaped the way that you practise and the way your business runs? We can listen and learn from your experience to improve experiences for those who may need our services, expertise or help in the future.

Sabia: Before I was a doula, I was in the medical field. I was a nursing assistant, on my way to becoming a nurse. I wanted to be a nurse practitioner. I knew I wanted to work in 'women's' health. That was all based on my desire to help people. I was in the medical field for around five years, but I quickly realized that all the disparities were based on race. We would have a lot of veterans come in and I was seeing a very clear difference between the black veterans' mental health and the white veterans' mental health. The black veterans' mental health would very much be post-traumatic stress disorder (PTSD) with severe symptoms. The white veterans would, largely, be in a much better place, physically and emotionally. That really sparked something in me. We were also really treating people in pieces. We would say, 'Oh you have this health condition, let me give you a pill', which might not be necessarily bad in some cases, but how can we give them a pill and not give them healthy food? How can we send them home without the education to help them get better? Or at least keep it where it is at and not get worse, right? I was seeing it so much. I didn't know if I wanted to be in the medical field anymore. Around that time, I heard about doulas and thought maybe that would be something closer to what I wanted to be able to do. With the work I was currently doing I didn't really feel like I had the space or time to dedicate myself to it, but it was still there in the back of my mind.

Every time I am at a crossroads or stress in my life like this it manifests itself in my body – that is just how my body works. I ended up having a heart problem, tachycardia. My heart rate would just randomly go up 30–40 beats per minute, even when I was just doing nothing. It put me out of work for two months. In that time, I made the decision that I was going to move. I took it as a sign that my heart was fucking up because I wasn't listening to it. So, I found the Prison Birth Project in Massachusetts and they were looking for volunteer doulas. I moved and started doing my training and working in the hospital too. I got my first client, and she was due in January 2016. I was so excited. I was doing antenatal education with my client from PBP (Prison Birth Project) and I was still working in the hospital. One day at work I started having this pain. It felt like my ribs were trying to move. It was this bizarre pain. I went to urgent care and told them what was going on. I had a white, male doctor. I told him all about the pain, told him it was not my usual. He wasn't really sure what to do, so he just sort of blurted out, 'Maybe it's your gallbladder?'

I said I hadn't ever had a problem with my gallbladder before so I wasn't sure if that was it. I wasn't saying it couldn't be my gallbladder, but it didn't seem right to me. He didn't palpate, he didn't put his hands on me or anything. He just gave me some medication and sent me to go about my business. I went back to work, then a few days later I went back to urgent care because something wasn't right. There was another white, male doctor. He said maybe it was kidney stones. Again, I've never had a problem with my kidneys or kidney stones before. Again, he didn't palpate me, he didn't do shit. Usually, they lie you down, have a feel about, right? None of that. At this point I had given up with the urgent care. I called my regular doctor and they got me in for later that week. I went to the appointment with my regular doctor, and he was an Indian guy, so a male, brown doctor. I told him what was going on, told him my experience. Lo and behold, he listened to me. He made me lie down, he palpated me, he said let's get a CAT scan – let's see what is going on.

He was the first person to touch me, to listen to me, to believe me and ask for further tests. During this time, I had become a new doula, I was teaching my client how to advocate for herself and here I was trying to advocate for myself. I was also realizing the benefits of having medical insurance, being a part of the medical world and knowing the terminology and the procedures. I finally got the CAT scan and I had a fibroid as big as my fist. It was pushing on my spine; it was pushing my uterus and bladder down causing all this pain. If I lay down on my side, you could literally feel it. If anyone had palpated me in the right position, they would have felt it right away. When I got the results, they said it was too big now so I needed surgery, but they couldn't do laparoscopic. It was now pretty much open abdominal surgery. I pushed the surgery back a bit so I could be with my client when she had her baby. I just made it; the baby was born a few days before my surgery. It was a close call! I ended up having complications from the surgery. It wasn't because they had done anything wrong, it was just scar tissue. That led to me having fibromyalgia and prob-lems with my pelvic floor. I then needed a second surgery a year later because my uterus had attached to my bowel. This is why I don't want to have children, why I don't want to carry children.

It's also a big part of why I am in this work. I imagine that if this was hard for me to navigate, as someone who is in that field and knows the terminology, how would other people do that? The part I always remember is that I went to so many doctors and they just didn't listen to me. They didn't listen. I was spelling it out for them, 'I have abdominal pain and all these symptoms', but they did not listen to me. It took until the third doctor, a brown doctor, to listen and try to figure it out. Even with my heart condition, the first doctor I saw told me I was just dehydrated; this was a white doctor. Then when I saw a brown doctor again, he listened and told me about my IST (inappropriate sinus tachycardia), and what he could do to help me. It really drove home the importance of having a doctor (or healthcare professional) who aligns with your identities. It literally saved my life. Twice.

There are further complications with aligning to my queer identity for me and my body that some healthcare professionals just wouldn't understand. They just can't. So how can they help me? Why can't I have doctors who understand these parts of my identity when it has been proven to be so important for my health? It is a big part of why I moved across the country to Atlanta because there are more black doctors there. There are more people who share intersections with me, so that when I am in their care, I can talk without having to explain every little thing about me. I don't have to explain everything to them. After those experiences, I have PTSD. So even thinking about pregnancy for me is just too much. The trust that I would have to put in the provider. The idea that I would not be in control of my body, especially in the US where we have created an environment and a culture where the doctors know your body better than you do. I can't do that, but I can be the person who helps others through that. That is what makes me good at what I do, because in some ways I have been there.

I created the birthing advocacy business specifically for those who are at the intersection of these various identities. I would look around the doula training schools and say, where is the care for the black people, the queer and trans people? There are so many ways that people exist, and you are just giving me the information to care for white, hetero, cis, upper class people. BADT (Birthing Advocacy Doula Trainings) was my answer to this missing space. It was clearly so needed because it's working and it's growing!

There is power in being aware of intersectionality. There is such power in being in the care of people who share your identities.

There is power in not having children if you don't want to have children.

*

Sabia is an absolute powerhouse in changing the care that marginalized folk expect and deserve from their care providers. Listening to her talking about her past experiences was hard, but a much-needed reminder that people from marginalized or oppressed groups walk through the systems and processes differently. It's a big reminder to always consider our intersectionality within our work. Go and do a BADT course; I promise it will change how you work.

Adoption: an interview with Kevin

When looking for people to talk with about adoption it can be quite tricky. There is the need for safety and anonymity for those who adopt. I spoke to Kevin, a pansexual dad of two adopted children. I asked him what he would like to tell healthcare professionals about families who grow their families through adoption.

AJ: This book isn't strictly for parents or expectant parents who are going through the processes of growing their family through adoption. It's more for the healthcare professionals who care for us, in the many ways that we exist; so, the health visitors, the doctors, midwives and so on. What do you, as a man in a same-sex relationship who adopted his children, want them to know?

Kevin: For me and my husband, this is the end of a very long journey. We started down the route of surrogacy first but that didn't work out for us. It cost us a hell of a lot of money, but as I say, it didn't work out.

Would you like me to talk about our experience of surrogacy as well as adoption?

AJ: Yes absolutely, you tell me what it is you want healthcare providers to know about your journey to becoming an LGBT+ parent.

Kevin: Sure, no problem. We used a private clinic, which we had to travel to. We live in a rural part of the country. We used an egg donor and a surrogate, so there were a lot of people involved. From a health-care professional's point of view, we weren't as involved as perhaps other parents would be. Questions were directed to the surrogate, or even her husband. He had to have counselling and he had to have a say in what was going on, but questions were very rarely directed at us. We felt really detached from the process. We sometimes just felt like the funders. With any decision or anything that was going on, we felt secondary to the process. The specialist would direct their discussion to the surrogate. First, they would make sure she was okay, rightly so, but then it was almost like we were secondary. Like we were not important. It was strange, quite a cold environment. It was very statistically driven; there was very little human element to it. We went through a miscarriage with our surrogate. Then we had a failed transfer of an embryo. All the discussion was with the surrogate; we really couldn't even ring up and ask to discuss what had happened because we weren't, on paper, involved with the baby. It made it so uncomfortable for us. When the surrogate had a miscarriage, we were in the dark about how she was and what was going on for over six hours. They just wouldn't discuss it with us on the phone. Of course, our concern was for the surrogate and how she was doing. We didn't want to be ringing her or her husband while she was going through this. However, we had also just lost our baby and we did feel we were very much on the outside, looking in.

AJ: How far removed the intended parents feel with the process has been quite a common theme with the other parents I have spoken to who have used donors or surrogates.

Kevin: Yes, exactly. Everything would be directed at the surrogate, then at the surrogate's husband. Then maybe, sometimes, they would say, 'Are you two okay with this?' It was an awkward situation to be in.

AJ: What is your ideal solution to that? How could healthcare professionals better involve intended parents in those processes? Would it be a case of honesty and saying something like, 'This is the deal. Legally speaking we must ask the surrogate for their permission. I hope you can understand that.' What else could it look like?

Kevin: Yes, I think because they were very directed questions. There were no open questions to the room. Obviously, we were four people involved in this situation, we had a very good relationship, we still do now. When we went for the scans, only one of us could go in. My husband went in, and I stayed in the waiting room with the surrogate's husband. That was another awkward situation. I don't know if it is just protocol to have two people in the room when having scans, but it really felt like the surrogate should have had who she wanted in there and that we, as the babies' dads, should also have been allowed in.

It just comes back down to the policies and the laws surrounding surrogacy really. Same-sex surrogacy isn't funded or recognized by the NHS. The laws need to change before the practices can change. The law and society aren't adjusting as quickly as families are. Families come in all shapes, sizes and existences and the policies just aren't there with us, yet.

AJ: I hear that! When I do my workshops and speak to healthcare professionals about how the policies can be harmful or restricting to families that don't exist within that assumed family structure, they understandably feel caught between a rock and a hard place. They must protect themselves and follow the procedures, but they also want to provide the best care that they can. Part of their allyship to LGBT+ families may involve being uncomfortable in saying to their superiors, 'I took care of a family yesterday and this policy doesn't work for them, because there are two mums or two dads or any other number of family structures that don't adhere to the cis heteronormative that our society assumes and expects.'

Kevin: Yeah, I agree! When we were told the first pregnancy was viable, we were planning where our surrogate would give birth. We are from different towns and different NHS trusts. We had to think about how that would happen. We were told following the birth of our baby that we wouldn't be allowed to walk out of the hospital with our baby. It would have to be the surrogate, 'the mum' as they said, to take the baby off the premises.

If there were difficulties in birth, so that 'mum had to stay in the hospital', then the baby had to stay in the hospital too. To us this felt as if it was totally in the Dark Ages. The NHS sells itself as being allied to the LGBT+ community, but it's just so, so far behind what other countries do for surrogacy families.

AJ: Yeah, we are so hugely behind North America, for example.

Kevin: Yeah, that is why so many people go to America for surrogacy, which is not assessable for everyone. In the UK, they just can't discuss anything with us directly. Even in our case where the surrogate isn't 'biologically linked'. We used a donor egg and my husband's sperm, and even then, we were just so often on the outside looking in.

AJ: That is a big part that often shocks people when it's discussed in my workshops; that even if the surrogate isn't biologically linked to the baby, the surrogate, and possibly even the surrogate's husband, will still be recorded as the mother and/or father on the birth certificate.

Kevin: Yeah, then it's a 12-week period to change it. So, parents are in limbo and then must adopt their own biological children.

AJ: People are so shocked by this.

Kevin: I don't blame the healthcare professionals in this, because obviously it's the policy and law makers.

AJ: Absolutely, of course. It is, however, a good example of how when you are making policies and procedures at any level you need to consider all types of families and situations, all types of people who will need these services. Then there are families that show up in these situations that haven't been considered and end up on the outside looking in, like you and your husband, and it becomes a case of 'computer says no' in some regards.

Kevin: Yes, but I'm not sure what the consequences would be if a doctor or midwife just said, 'This policy obviously doesn't apply to you because you are two dads', or whatever, if they tried to fit the policies round the families, rather than the families round the policies.

AJ: Yes! That's the ideal situation, isn't it? That everyone can give the care they want to and are able to give. Fit the policies round the family and not the families round the policies.

Kevin: Yep, that is what doesn't happen. When you go down the adoption route, you get assigned all these different social workers. Where we live, it's quite a rural area, and so same-sex adoption isn't as common. They do these courses, every few months, for adoptive parents. We were the only same-sex couple on there. The social workers for want of a better word were...older women, 'traditional' older women. One of them even started to discuss breastfeeding with my husband. She was just so used to talking to heterosexual couples and was on autopilot a bit I suppose. It took her a while to catch up to what she was saying. She was talking about skin-to-skin contact as well, then cut herself off short saying, 'Well, you can't do skin-to-skin either.'

AJ: Why couldn't you do skin-to-skin?

Kevin: Well, our children were removed at birth, but they were taken into emergency foster care. We could have done foster to adopt, but there is always a chance that a judge will decide that they should go back with their birth family. That wasn't something that we could put ourselves through. Bonding with a baby at birth, then having them taken away. We had already suffered through loss with surrogacy, and we just, just couldn't do it.

AJ: Yeah, I see.

Kevin: Our children had no skin-to-skin contact when they were born. It stayed that way because they were premature. So, when they were taken out of hospital by foster carers, we were made aware. They hound it into you all the way through that this might not work out. They might not come to live with you. They always tell you to prepare for the worse, well the worst for you. The most important thing is what is best for the children, so if it's best to stay with their birth mum then that is what will happen. If it's best for the children to be adopted by a family that will love them, then that is what will happen. You have to put a lot of faith in the system.

We have nothing but empathy for our children's birth mum. We have met her as well, and we did that so that when the children are older, we can tell them: we've met her, this is what she was like and this was the situation and why you didn't live with her.

We can't not be open because we're two cis men.

AJ: Yep, that makes sense.

Kevin: Going back to the professionals for a minute. When we were dealing with the social workers, their courses, forms and all that stuff was completely in the wrong language for us. Everything is just geared towards this nuclear family ideal. The social worker just couldn't move past that we were two men sometimes. She kept coming back to the reports you must do when you adopt. Social services must go to your ex-partners and anyone you have ever lived with to talk to them, rightly so, to check you out, check there was no abuse or anything going on. I have ex-girlfriends and ex-boyfriends. She kept coming back to my sexuality all the time, asking when I stopped being straight and started being gay. I told her you can't keep asking these questions. She said, 'So are you bi then?' It was just exhausting. I don't label myself too strictly, but if I did, I would be closer to pan(sexual) than anything else, but then she had to google what pan was, so I don't think that really helped her understand it.

AJ: Oh my god, I feel for you as a fellow pansexual. I have known so many people who have had to google pansexual when I talk to them about it. This really ties into the Stonewall *LGBT+ in Britain* report that tells us that 'One in four LGBT+ people have experienced inappropriate curiosity from healthcare staff because they are LGBT.'[12]

Kevin: That was my biggest bugbear throughout the whole process. Rightly so, they must go back and make sure you are safe for these babies or children. I get it. The social worker just had a field day with my exes. Not because there are loads of them but because there were people of different genders and sexualities on there too. She tended to hover around the subject, especially when she met my family members. My dad is quite a traditional guy, not down with talking about these sorts of things, especially with people he's just met. The social worker seemed to really want to 'dig' into this part of my life. It almost felt like it was a bit of research into my sexual preferences and not really anything else.

AJ: How is your sexuality or sexual history relevant to how good a dad you would be?

Kevin: Well, exactly. I don't know if she was trying to suggest that maybe I am easily changed, or I don't stick with something? I honestly don't know. My husband and I have been together eight years and

12 www.stonewall.org.uk/system/files/lgbt_in_britain_health.pdf

my previous relationship before that was six years, with a woman. I just think it might have been a generational thing. In fact, I sent the social worker a resource, like a wheel of fortune, and the spaces on the wheel are populated with different genders and sexualities, and when the wheel stops you must explain what that means or what that is.

AJ: That sounds amazing!

Kevin: She said she used it in the office with the other social workers! Which is good I suppose, but I did think I shouldn't have to do this. I shouldn't have to explain all of this to you.

AJ: It should never be the place of LGBT+ people to explain all of this to people, to anyone, while we are in such a vulnerable place in our lives.

Kevin: Uh-huh, no.

AJ: So that was the social worker, who maybe needs to read this book, or go on a workshop or something. Tell me about any other healthcare professionals you saw. Was there an awesome health visitor who just got it? Was there a GP who didn't assume anything? Tell me about everyone else.

Kevin: We didn't have midwives come to visit because the children were seven weeks when they came to us, so they were discharged from midwife care by that point. We had health visitors that came to see us. We also went to the local weigh-in clinic as well.

I don't know if I am being hypersensitive, but, when the health visitors would tell us how to care for the children, they were quite, um, what is the best word, thorough? I don't know if it was because we were two men. They maybe thought that we might not have been as good or know as much as a heterosexual couple or a woman would have done. There wasn't anything they specifically said or did, but just the way it felt, was that they were going over it again because we were blokes.

We have had a couple comments, where healthcare professionals or general people have said to us, 'I wish my husband was as good with my children as you are with yours', stuff along that line. Maybe they are insinuating that we are better with kids because we are gay? We get it quite a lot at like toddler groups and stuff like that. When we do go to these groups, we do feel like they are overly, like, helpful? Trying to make sure we can do it. There is this aspect of maybe people think we can't do it. Or there is this lower expectation of what we can do because we are men.

AJ: The patriarchal assumption that men aren't as good as raising children as women harms us all!

Kevin: Yes! Absolutely.

AJ: This assumption that someone will be a better parent because of their shell, because of their body, can be harmful.

Kevin: It's the assumption, isn't it? When we go to appointments sometimes, they've obviously read the notes and know that these children have two dads, but sometimes they haven't. There has only been one occasion where a doctor asked me, 'Where is Mum?', and I took great delight in telling the doctor, 'My children have two dads.'

We are due to get the children's birth certificate back soon. The one with our family name on it, as at the moment it has their surname at birth on there. It was asked if we wanted to have a 'celebration day'. Sometimes they offer this 'special' ceremony that they do to 'officially' give you the birth certificate. My husband and I have a bit of an issue with this really, because it's a bit sad. It's a bit sad that the boys have 'lost' their other family. We write to their birth family twice a year to let them know how they are growing up and getting on and all that. These celebration days can seem a bit tokenistic. Maybe it's meant to replace a christening or something. It just feels a bit wrong. Of course, we are happy to have these documents but it's not like a 'victory' to celebrate for us.

Also, we were meant to have these (birth certificates) within ten weeks, but it's nearly two years down the road now. They are nearly two and still have the surname that was given to them at birth. That is their birth dad's surname. He's never seen them. Never had any contact or wanted any contact with them. It does kind of grieve us that we must keep this surname even though we are their dads.

Anyone going through this process should know that it is such a long road. They say it takes six months, this new streamlined process, but it just doesn't happen like that. Our local authority has an advert saying, 'Apply to adopt now and you could be on the beach with your kids in the summer!' It's just so unrealistic and really sets people up for heartache.

AJ: Yeah, that doesn't sound possible at all, does it? Surely all these checks and forms are going to take much longer than that.

Kevin: Yes, of course they will.

AJ: On the new birth certificates, will you be listed as parent one and parent two?

Kevin: Do you know what? That is a good question. I don't know. On the ones we have now it's mother and father. I am not sure how it will look.

AJ: In some instances, with same-sex parents I have worked with, if they are married then they can go down as parent one and parent two.

Kevin: We won't both be down as father, I know that much. Thinking back to how we've been treated when dealing with healthcare professionals in the past, I've never been asked, 'How do you want to be referred to? What should I call you in relation to your children?' Usually what happens is they are waiting for us to use a name for each other. If I say to the children 'Go to Daddy' or 'Come to Dad' then they start using that terminology, which is obviously great and fine. But they should be asking us, so we don't have to try and let them know what we want to be called or what we are called to our kids. They should be able to ask straightaway.

AJ: Yes, asking these open questions like 'Who have you brought with you today?' That is one that I get a lot as a doula when I am with a family at appointments or at birth. It's usually an obstetrician or midwife who comes into the room and they see the birthing person over there, someone else who is the dad or the partner or whatever, then they are looking at me, thinking, 'Who the fuck are you!', and that is okay, I don't mind that. They will say something diplomatic like 'Shall we go around the room and introduce ourselves?' when really all they want to know is, who the fuck I am. In those circumstances, they are totally okay with asking me who I am, probably as I am read as a cis woman, so maybe the birthing person's sister or, maybe in a few years, their mother, or something. In those circumstances, they are okay with it, so why can't they do that with all the families that come through? Ask, nicely, who is here with us today, who have you brought with you today, rather than assuming a family's make up is based on cis heteronormativity.

Kevin: It never happens with pronouns either. I am a teacher and I make sure to ask all my students their pronouns. I never want to get it wrong and put someone in a position where they must come to me and explain or out themselves.

In an ideal world with the birth certificate, it wouldn't be parent one and parent two. Everyone would be able to say how they want to be recorded, for their actual relationship with the baby.

I would hope that none of my children would shout 'Parent two, can you come help me?' at the park or anything. I would see that as quite cold terminology really. Also, who is going to be parent two?!

AJ: You would never hear 'parent two' at the park!

Kevin: I've never thought of it before, it's quite thought provoking!

AJ: I am so glad I could come and give you something else to be angry about on a Saturday afternoon!

Kevin: [laughing] Oh no, not at all. It just never occurred to me before you said it. This is amazing, it's like therapy for me to be able to tell you all of this.

AJ: Well, that's kind. It's so important to have these discussions. I have never, yet, spoken to any healthcare professional and they've said that they are outwardly homophobic, or transphobic. They always say how much they want to be able to support us and help us. But because it's so seldom talked about or discussed, without knowing it, they aren't prepared and can hurt us.

Kevin: Just asking would be the sensible thing to do. Asking these questions about who we are, what we want to be called, our biological relationship to the baby, our emotional relationship with the baby. Just ask so we can tell you best how to refer to us. We live in this society where people are genuinely terrified of offending people, using the wrong words and so on.

AJ: Oh brother, yes. That is one of the big things that we need to talk about. We need to be sure that we can tell people, particularly the people who care for our health, how they can do that as best as possible.

Kevin: I think that tends to get lost a bit with healthcare professionals, because they are so rushed and underfunded. That human element just gets lost a bit. The government, as well, needs to make the changes at the highest levels so they can filter down. Realistically, no one can make changes until the government tells them to, or gives them the resources to change it, the time, and the money. When it comes to applying for anything, the forms and what have you, it's so prevalent, isn't it? This assumption of heteronormativity. When we applied for the adoption order the forms literally said: adoptive mum and adoptive dad. Even with the reading lists that came with the adoption courses, so few even mentioned same-sex parents or the differences and difficulties of same-sex adoption. I've never seen anything written about these pitfalls before. Even just hearing someone else talk about the assumptions or difficulties with doctors or health visitors would have been nice. Thinking about that beforehand just adds this layer of stress and worry about how your life will be if you finally get a child placed with you. Being able to read about other people's experiences and stories would have been so helpful, as I am sure they are for the heterosexual parents who read the books on the reading list. Parents are all so different; even within my relationship, my husband is so different from me. When someone asks me where our children's mum is, I'll tell them that they have two dads, but my husband says, 'She's at work.' He is just so averse to the possible conflict that could arise that he finds it better to lie.

AJ: Oh wow, that's horrible. I don't mean it's horrible he does that, whatever works for you, I mean that he feels he must lie.

Kevin: We could make it awkward for people, couldn't we? 'Where is their mum?' We could say, 'Dunno, haven't seen her for a while.'

AJ: Oh gosh, could you imagine?!

Kevin: But we don't want people to feel awkward around us!

AJ: It reminds me of when people ask childless people, 'When are you having kids?' There could be something happening in their life, with their health, or anything like that. They may just not want kids. Why do people have to ask these horrific closed questions? It happens to independent parents too. I am trying to train myself out of saying single parents as not all parents are single and that implies that they were coupled, and some parents are just independent of a couple.

When people ask 'Where is Mummy?' or 'Where is Daddy?' and you are asking a child of an independent parent, how will that go down?

Kevin: That is one thing that IVF taught us. It is a miracle that anyone gets pregnant when you go through the system from this side of it. The chances can seem so small.

You just cannot assume anything about families and how they are made. Saying that, some of the newer social workers that we have had are better with the terminology and knowing what to say and what not to say to a same-sex family. I think there is change starting and it is going to make the process so much better for so many people.

AJ: Yes, I think it is changing, slowly, but we must push forward to change the system and the people in it too.

Kevin: I don't understand why it is so difficult in this country for two people to come together and have a family. That is what tends to get lost. There are a lot of cis men and cis women who aren't together and co-parent. I don't understand why it must be such an issue. The top and bottom of the issue is, children need love, from one or more people. It doesn't matter what their gender or sexuality. That is all it comes down to.

*

Amen Kevin, amen.

Risk: does a medicalized conception mean a medicalized birth?

Many parents, not just LGBT+ parents who have a medicalized conception, may feel worried or restricted due to the assumption or insistence that they need a medicalized birth. IVF pregnancies are often treated as high risk from the outset.[13]

---

13 www.nice.org.uk/guidance/cg156/chapter/Recommendations

Risks of twins and multiples are increased with IVF when implanting more than one embryo;[14] however, IUI (in utero insemination – the act of inserting sperm into the womb) doesn't show an increased likelihood of multiples.[15]

Multiple births aside, many of the risks, or perceived risks, from assisted pregnancies can come from underlying conditions which may have been the cause of the infertility in the first place.[16] We must ask, for families whose fertility issue is simply that they don't have the biology between them to make a baby, does this increase risk?

So often, as a birth worker who spends their days talking to other birth workers, and indeed as a gestational parent myself in the past, I hear that it's about policy. That is how it works here. You have/ are XYZ so that means you must do XYZ. Until I read the AIMS publication *Am I Allowed*,[17] I wasn't aware of the extent of some of the negatives of generalized care. So many parents are expected to fit into boxes that fit the best for them. Fat? High risk. Assisted pregnancy? High risk. Previous caesarean section? High risk. The really maddening thing is that in one trust you may be high risk for something that your mate down the road, three miles away, under a different hospital with the same 'high-risk marker', isn't high risk.

These processes and procedures can be frustrating for parents and for the healthcare professionals themselves. It often goes further than being slightly annoying for many parents. It could increase risk.

Take my experience for a moment, as I believe it is an excellent example of how wide, generalized, sweeping policies can increase risk for pregnant people.

When I was pregnant in 2015 with my second child, I was told that because I had gestational diabetes previously, I would again be placed on a high-risk pathway. I declined this level of care, as I was going to birth Emma at home. I knew that going onto a consultant-led

---

14   www.nhs.uk/conditions/ivf/risks
15   www.fertilityiq.com/iui-or-artificial-insemination/how-well-iui-works-by-patient-type#defining-iui-success
16   www.nice.org.uk/guidance/cg156/chapter/Recommendations
17   www.aims.org.uk/general/am-i-allowed

pathway would make it less likely I would be 'granted' a home birth, despite the right to choose where we give birth being written into Department of Health policy and European Union human rights. The Department of Health's guidance[18] stated that choice of where to give birth, including home birth, was a national choice guarantee.

However, in making my choice of where to give birth, I was told that I would still have to see the consultant, have extra scans, more appointments and see the diabetes midwife. I had been given information on gestational diabetes in my first pregnancy three years earlier and I still had my testing kit. I reassured the midwife that I was already monitoring my sugars when I went to my booking appointment and said I would let them know if I needed any support or further input. This did seem to satisfy my consultant who was nice enough to give me a letter to 'allow' my home birth. First-time parents, or indeed parents who are already 'high risk' for other reasons such as BMI, method of conception or all manner of otherings, may not have this knowledge or even the ability to stand their ground to fight for their birth choices. I was lucky that I had support from my spouse and other birth workers.

Some LGBT+ parents may feel safer to give birth at home, whether this is because they are concerned for their safety, gender/sexuality assumptions, worried about making others uncomfortable if they are masculine presenting in an often assumed to be exclusively feminine environment, and more. Whatever the parents' thought process or justification, it is the eternal hope that individualized care and continuity of care can be given to enable each person to make their own informed decision on what is right for them and for their baby.

BMI

Of all the things that can get in the way, BMI is a big one for me. Body mass index, invented 200 or so years ago, using only cis, white

---

18 https://webarchive.nationalarchives.gov.uk/20130103004823/http://www.dh.gov. uk/en/Publicationsandstatistics/Publications/PublicationsPolicyAndGuidance/ DH_073312

men as a basis,[19] is often completely arbitrary to say the least. I have supported families where the mother was 31 on the BMI scale. (A healthy BMI as quantified by the NHS is 18.5–25; overweight is 25–30, and 30 and over is obese.[20]) A woman who cycled several miles to work a day, who swam into her 41st week of pregnancy, ate food from her garden and walked frequently in the woods with her dogs, when having her weight recorded at her 12-week booking appointment, was told, as her BMI was over 30, that she would be high risk. Thankfully, when she saw the consultant, the consultant was rather frustrated that she had been referred and signed it all off to be cared for back in the community. The point is that sweeping policies seldom work for everyone. Some elements of individualized care and thought need to go into referrals and policy. This isn't often compatible with the NHS; however, when considering LGBT+ families, extra consideration may need to be given to the actual cause of the high-risk status. Is this woman or pregnant person at an increased risk due to XYZ, or is this just how we have always done it?

Unknown donor

The primary question I pose to healthcare professionals when discussing this is: 'Is this situation any different to a cis or hetero parent falling pregnant after sex with an anonymous partner?' I spoke to Adelaide Harris, a registered midwife working within the NHS in London, and this is what she told me:

> The position around IVF pregnancies varies around the country. The Royal College of Obstetricians and Gynaecologists' scientific impact paper was published 2012[21] and states that, overall, most IVF pregnancies have good outcomes. Poorer outcomes inevitably reflect aspects of the treatment but also the interplay with the underlying features that the couple bring to the pregnancy.

---

19 www.ncbi.nlm.nih.gov/pmc/articles/PMC2930234
20 www.nhs.uk/live-well/healthy-weight/bmi-calculator
21 www.rcog.org.uk/en/guidelines-research-services/guidelines/?q=&subject=&-type=Scientific+Impact+Papers&orderby=title

The advice is that a risk assessment and appropriate referral are key. I would argue that this is true for any pregnancy.

The NHS is a gift, there is no doubt about it. The challenge of having free at point of access care is that it requires several systems and structures to enable a universal standard of care for a large scale. Working in a case-loading model allows me to consider the individual needs of each family. Case-loading care requires more time, more midwives and a flexibility in structure that organizations are currently in the process of adapting. There is no possible way that we could care for the volume of people that we do without more resources – time, staff, facilities.

Guidelines are advice on best practice. The frequency with which they are updated may mean that there is newest evidence available that is not integrated into national guidance until the next version is published. The best care relies on midwives and other healthcare professionals being able to source the most relevant research to support out-of-guidance birth. When guidance isn't presented as a choice, the onus is put on the pregnant person and their family to navigate through the system and unpack the recommendations.

Pregnancy and birth are not without risks. Eventually we must ask ourselves the question, when does the impact of intervention outweigh the risks that they are trying to mitigate? With inductions and caesarean sections rising in number, we must be under no illusions as to the impact that it has on birth experience as well as future pregnancies.

The language I prefer is complex care. Some may say that it is not a question of language, but language has power. It's why we're advised to use chance instead of risk when talking about antenatal screening.

I'm not an expert and have had no experience 'assisting' or coaching a free birther. Free birthing is a legitimate choice, yet I have encountered some people who express a desire to have an unassisted birth because of the fear of medicalization or the lack of control that they have previously experienced in their birthing environment. I accept that everyone can make any choice that is right for them, but I feel uncomfortable with choices that are made when motivated by fear alone. This relates to all aspects of care throughout the childbirth continuum.

Iatrogenesis is a topic worthy of a book of its own. As Sara Wickham says:

> The iatrogenic effects of health care, according to Ivan Illich, come in a variety of forms from clinical iatrogenesis, where medical intervention causes side effects which are worse than the original problem, to social and structural iatrogenesis, which describe states where people become docile and reliant on the medical profession and/or give up their autonomy.[22, 23]

BMI is a good example of this. Body weight stigma is perpetuated under the guise of health. The idea that your weight alone is an indicator of health doesn't make a lot of sense to me. Being in a bigger body, having a higher BMI, brings limitations on birth choices.[24] This makes me wonder if poorer outcomes are increased because of restricted access to home birth, birth centres and increased surveillance in the form of ultrasound scans and continuous monitoring. Cardiotocography monitoring increases the risk of caesarean section.

Fundamentally, an unknown donor makes no difference. Not only that, but unless we have full access to GP records, we are always relying on a person's recollection and perception of their own and their family's medical history. It's why surveillance and screening throughout pregnancy to identify signs of developing complexities is important.

Mental health in pregnancy isn't my area of speciality, but I

22 www.sarawickham.com/riffing-ranting-and-raving/fear-of-childbirth-or-fear-of-medicalisation

23 www.sarawickham.com/quotes-and-shares/quote-of-the-month-for-august-the-balance-sheet-of-risk

24 *My Fat Friend: The Bizarre and Racist History of BMI*: https://elemental.medium.com/the-bizarre-and-racist-history-of-the-bmi-7d8dc2aa33bb

think emotional risk and mental wellbeing in pregnancy sit side by side. We can talk about birth trauma statistics – about 30,000 people a year suffer from birth trauma.[25] We could also link this to what usually causes trauma – lack of control, feelings of helplessness and so on.

What we are pushing back against is a system which still assumes that all pregnancies are the result of cis heteronormative relationships. Or, worse, a system that recognizes that not all families conform to the presumed default but the numbers are not big enough to be worth making changes that would include and affirm them. The organizational and structural barriers of computer systems and paperwork prevent recognition of family constellations which don't fit into this mould. Not being recognized by the healthcare system can impact on the commissioning of care and provision of professional education programmes that meet the needs of LGBT+ families.

Simple acts of kindness are often displayed by individuals but are not representative of the healthcare system as a whole.

What do you do when there isn't space and time for the pregnant person to tell you what they need to tell you? Midwives feel this frustration so acutely. As someone working in a continuity model, I know that it is a privilege to be able to give each pregnant person the space and time required for them to feel heard. Not everyone is as proactive or knows enough about what a booking appointment entails to be able to request a longer appointment. My heart sinks when I'm covering booking clinics and a person answers my question asking them about themselves and their medical history with 'How long have you got?' I'm thinking about the next person in the waiting room, the lunch break I can work through or the clinic I'm covering. When I recognize that a person may need more time than I have available for them, I think about how best I can use the time we do have to get to know them in a way that builds rapport and may allow for a more expedient

---

25 www.birthtraumaassociation.org.uk/#

follow-up appointment where I can fill in the required boxes. This may also include performing screening tests as appropriate. Overall, my focus is about the experience as this sets the tone and expectation for the remaining care. It suits no one when appointments are rushed or when questions are asked and the answers are only listened to for the correct box to be ticked.

I'm not sure if I want to say that closed questions are asked intentionally, if unconsciously, due to time constraints. It's like when I worked as a member of a cabin crew and used to stride down the aisle with my eyeline raised so that no one could use eye contact to catch my attention and ask for something.

For clinical midwives, it can feel very difficult to make significant changes to the way that services are delivered. When we try, we are confronted with the harsh reality that NHS trusts also are businesses. When the operational needs overshadow the quality of care, we must push back against those constraints. It can be unnerving when everyone else is going with the flow, and not questioning why there isn't more time available. 'That's just the way it is' is the answer to many a question asked, but is that good enough?

When discussing risk, we cannot ignore emotional or financial risk. When we are talking about clinical risk, we often have statistics to prove that there is a higher likelihood of a negative or detrimental impact or outcome due to these differences or difficulties. Emotional risk cannot be quantified as easily. With so many parents and well-meaning others still trotting out old and harmful tropes such as 'All that matters is a healthy baby' it's no wonder that so many people compromise with a process that is presented as the only way to be safe.

CHAPTER 6

Perinatal Mental Health

When thinking about what on earth I could cite or back up with statistics in this chapter, I am so lucky to know Dr Mari Greenfield, who works at King's College London. They are also a queer doula, and a dear friend. They have worked tirelessly and diligently in their field for decades, using their skills and time to aid in research, funding requests and results for the LGBT+ community of parents and birth workers in the UK. Mari has first had experience of LGBT+ parenting, as a foster parent and birthing their own children. Mari lives in the north of England with her family. Mari uses they/them and she/her pronouns.

Mari was kind enough to share some of their recent research that they have done with Zoe Darwin into trans and non-binary pregnancy, traumatic birth and perinatal mental health.[1]

The report starts by, rightly, pointing out that many countries don't record data on gender in perinatal services. In fact, Australia is the only country that does so! Trying to discuss, fix or implement changes to improve outcomes for an already at-risk group of people is impossible without collecting this data in the first place. Does your trust or business collect this data? If not, how will there ever be visibility, change or improvement for communities which we know already face disparities in the wider world? Greenfield and Darwin's article goes on to explain that as the wider transgender population

---

1   Greenfield, M. and Darwin, Z. (2020) 'Trans and non-binary pregnancy, traumatic birth and perinatal mental health: A scoping review.' *International Journal of Transgender Health*, 22(1–2), pp. 203–216, doi: 10.1020/26895269.2020.1841057

already (outside the perinatal period) experiences higher rates of mental health difficulties and suicidality, this could indicate a higher likelihood of perinatal mental health (PMH) difficulties. Any parent can experience PMH difficulties; however, predisposing factors include a history of mental illness, trauma or abuse, lack of social support and poor care. Therefore, it is reasonable to expect a higher prevalence of PMH difficulties in the LGBT+ community, which is more likely to have predisposing factors.

PMH difficulties impact between 10 and 20 per cent of cisgender (cis) women.[2] In addition, an estimated 8 per cent of fathers experience postnatal depression.[3] The Birth Trauma Association tells us that an estimated 30 per cent of birthing parents in the UK experience some symptoms of PTSD.[4] Trans populations are disproportionately affected by violence[5] and other forms of trauma.

The prevalence of PMH difficulties and traumatic birth in trans and non-binary parents is unknown, because trans identities are so seldom captured. However, considering all that we know about cis women and men who experience PMH difficulties and what puts them at a higher statistical risk of this, we can draw a reasonable conclusion that trans and non-binary people giving birth and parenting are at a heightened risk of suffering with poor PMH.

Greenfield and Darwin's report concludes that:[6]

Existing literature suggests factors such as dysphoria, isolation and exclusion, and poor care may make trans and non-binary parents more vulnerable to PMH difficulties and traumatic birth.

---

2   https://www.gov.uk/government/publications/better-mental-health-jsna-toolkit/4-perinatal-mental-health

3   Cameron, E.E., Sedov, I.D and Tomfohr-Madsen, L.M. (2016) 'Prevalence of paternal depression in pregnancy and the postpartum: An updated meta-analysis.' *Journal of Affective Disorders*, 206, pp. 189–203, doi: 10.1016/j.jad.2016.07.044

4   https://www.birthtraumaassociation.org.uk/for-health-professional/supporting-parents-with-birth-trauma

5   Lombardi, E.L., Wilchins, R.A., Priesing, D. and Malouf, D. (2002) 'Gender Violence: Transgender Experiences with Violence and Discrimination.' *Journal of Homosexuality*, 42(1), pp. 89–101, doi: 10.1300/J082v42n01_05

6   Greenfield and Darwin (2020) p. 214

However, trans and non-binary parents' PMH experience remain under-researched. There are indications that without better information and awareness amongst parents and professionals, there may be distinct barriers to identifying PMH needs and accessing relevant support.

Without the ability to accurately record gender data within perinatal services, robust assessments of prevalence rates and longevity of specific diagnosable conditions will remain difficult to obtain; potential inequalities will remain hidden, and the ability to adapt services to meet local needs will be limited. Voices of trans and non-binary people are needed in PMH research to inform future services and improve outcomes for all parents and families.

What about perinatal mental health outcomes for same-sex families? Knowing what we know now from Greenfield and Darwin's report, we can quite safely assume that same-sex couples would also fall into some of the same categories for increased risk. Looking at the wider LGBT+ community, we know the increased risk of isolation and increased risk associated with the myriad of disparities faced by LGBT+ people, health, social and emotional.

Yana Sigal wrote 'Perinatal mental health in same-sex female couples' at the University of Pennsylvania in 2009.' Yana stated in the abstract for this piece, similarly to trans and non-binary parents and the findings of Greenfield and Darwin's report: 'Perinatal depression and increased stress levels may be more prevalent in same-sex female couples than heterosexually active couples.'

Several studies have illustrated that lesbians are at greater risk for heightened stress and anxiety around the time of pregnancy and family planning.[8] Improved education for healthcare professionals may lead to greater awareness of how to cater to alternative families. Simple changes like using gender neutral words such as 'partner'

7   https://repository.upenn.edu/cgi/viewcontent.cgi?article=1012&context=josnr
8   Trettin S., Moses-Kolko E.L. and Wisner K.L. (2006) 'Lesbian perinatal depression and the heterosexism that affects knowledge about this minority population.' *Arch Womens Ment Health*, 9(2), pp. 67–73, doi: 10.1007/s00737-005-0106-8

or 'significant other' instead of 'father of the baby', 'boyfriend' or 'husband' can make a safer atmosphere for lesbian couples. Creating a comfortable environment for same-sex female couples can lead to disclosure of sexual orientation, which provides information for the healthcare professional on how to provide the best service for these couples, ensure optimum care and decrease the risk of perinatal depression within this population.

When looking for studies or any information on the experience of cis men in same-sex relationships, I found within the *Journal of Reproductive and Infant Psychology* an article called 'Mothers and others: The invisibility of LGBTQ people in reproductive and infant psychology'.[9] Research into gay men's experiences of parenting through surrogacy has focused on the children's developmental outcomes, and the complex politics of surrogacy. No research focusing on gay men's experiences of or involvement in the actual surrogate pregnancy and birth has been undertaken, and information on the new fathers' perinatal mental health is scarce.

We know, from Greenfield and Darwin's 2020 review (above), that 5–15 per cent of cis fathers experience perinatal depression and anxiety. Using what we know are factors that increase cisgender and heterosexual parents' likelihood of experiencing poor perinatal mental health difficulties, we can, again, comfortably draw the assumption that cis men in same-sex relationships are likely to be at increased risk of PMH difficulties.

When we further consider minority stress of all the othered intersectional members of the LGBT+ community, it is easy to see how the cascading risk flows between these communities.

Mari Greenfield – perinatal mental health within the LGBT+ community

I first met Mari through a doula organization when they shared some of their research in a Facebook group. Through mutual interest and a shared kinship of LGBT+ identities, a friendship formed.

---

9   www.tandfonline.com/doi/full/10.1080/02646838.2019.1649919

Having watched Mari work as a researcher and a doula for years, I knew they were the best person to speak to about perinatal mental health within the LGBT+ community.

Mari: I think we need to break it down into different bits, PMH isn't just one thing. Yes, LBT people have greater risk of previous trauma, which can set them up for having PMH difficulties. But, if you want to look at something specific like birth trauma, which is my area, there are three things that interact. The first is previous life history – which includes things like domestic abuse, previous sexual abuse, experiences of rape or sexual abuse as an adult – existing mental health conditions, and existing substance abuse problems, including problematic drug use, not just drug use. All those things are somewhat tied together. You are more likely to have an underlying mental health problem if you are a victim of domestic violence. We know that black women are more likely to experience a traumatic birth, and the mechanism is assumed to be a lifetime of living with racism and microaggressions. There is an argument that would also apply to a lifetime of living with homophobia or transphobia.

The second part of what makes a birth traumatic is the actual event of the birth itself. You are more likely to have a traumatic birth if you have lots of medical intervention, particularly if those are outside your control.

The third thing is the care that you receive during labour. In terms of the events during labour, we don't have any data. We don't collect sexuality or gender identity data. We just don't know what is happening. There is a suspicion that lesbians are more likely to give birth when they are older and that makes it more likely to have interventions. The care received is likely to include homophobia and transphobia.

AJ: Would it also be fair to suggest that lesbians and same-sex couples assigned female at birth having conceived through home insemination, IUI or IVF are more likely to have intervention-heavy births?

Mari: Well, that is certainly true of IVF, but I don't think it's true of IUI. It depends on why the IVF was needed. If it is for an actual fertility problem, then those interventions may be appropriate. Sometimes it can come down to a problem of routing. What pathway or care plan you are put into because of the method of conception? The NICE guidelines state that you shouldn't be put on a high-risk pathway because of IVF alone. So, it's a matter of ignorance sometimes.

AJ: Yes, that has been a theme of the experiences of LGBT+ couples who have used IVF, IUI or AI (artificial insemination). If they are conceiving through IVF, IUI or AI because neither person has any sperm, should that be means of automatic high-risk status?

Mari: Yes, and then there is an assumption from healthcare professionals that when you talk about assisted conception you are talking about IVF. This could be DIY at home. It may or may not include sex. Sometimes people will talk about a donor because that is the role of that person in the family, but the method of conception will be sexual intercourse, the same as most heterosexual couples. Sometimes it won't include sexual intercourse, but that isn't IUI either, it's not the same. We don't know if that increases risk. Does it damage sperm?

AJ: Is it any different from people falling pregnant through transfer of sperm after ejaculation outside penetrative, penis-in-vagina sex? Is there a difference between home insemination for same-sex couples vs het folks who fall pregnant after sperm transfer?

Mari: We just don't know.

AJ: Would a cis heteronormative person necessarily think to divulge to a healthcare professional, who they might not even know, how they fell pregnant? That was another thing I was mulling over recently. It's impossible to look at this, though, because there is no paper trail to examine the differences between outcomes.

Mari: No, the data has just not been captured. What we do know, not from research but from lesbian self-help manuals and the like, is that certain types of plastic, which are used as receptacles, can damage sperm, but the research is just not there.

Another part of the paper was that gender dysphoria should be considered a specific PMH diagnosis. Even in non-binary people who hadn't experienced gender dysphoria beforehand, the evidence indicated that gender dysphoria could become a mental health issue during pregnancy. It really seemed to depend on whether their dysphoria was rooted internally or in the social aspect.

AJ: Yes of course, because some cis women experience body dysmorphia in pregnancy.

Mari: That is incredibly common. It seems to be connected to people who have tokophobia (pathological fear of pregnancy) and cis women who have hormonal dysphoria.

AJ: I think that is such a pertinent point. A lot of my time is spent explaining to people that improving understanding, awareness and practices around issues for LGBT+ people would improve outcomes and experiences for non-LGBT+ people also.

Mari: Yes, for cis women and trans folk it can go both ways. It is important to note that for cis women and trans folk alike, pregnancy can also be the time they feel most comfortable in their skin.

AJ: Yes, that is important.

Mari: Another issue is that sexual orientation is not included in any maternity statistics. Even Australia, which does capture data on gender identity, doesn't capture it. My Covid research has accidently become the biggest ever study of pregnant lesbian and bisexual women in the UK. It is not because it is something I set out to do, it's just because I asked the question. Seventy-six people out of 1700 were queer. We're not even up at the 10 per cent range and yet it's become the biggest study. Because nobody asks.

AJ: Wow.

Mari: In an article we wrote in the *Journal of Reproductive and Infant Psychology*,[10] Zoe and I reckon that there is a 10 per cent year on year growth of LGBT+ people accessing maternity and perinatal services.

AJ: We know there is a 20 per cent increase year on year of lesbians registering babies as well, don't we?

Mari: Yes, that's in the article I am talking about. This shouldn't have been the biggest study of queers in maternity, it just shouldn't have been. It's ridiculous. I don't understand why nowhere else is asking for LGBT+ status. It is interesting to look at the census too. We are going to have questions that ask about gender identity now, but still not sexuality.

AJ: It does seem backward. When I have a look at studies like those by Stonewall, they often break it down to lesbians, bisexuals, non-binary, trans, disabled, black and brown people in the statistics and you can very quickly see the disparities between these groups. There are a lot of people who are using maternity and perinatal services who are 'written off' as they are in invisible LGBT+ relationships or assumed to be in non-LGBT+ relationships. For example, all my data would have been assumed to be a cis het woman. So, when you start to look at the statistics of mental health, addiction, isolation, it's usually bisexual people who top the charts, so to speak. Therefore, at booking appointments and so on, if making assumptions about someone's sexuality based on who their partner(s) is or are, healthcare professionals may miss that a person is at increased risk of PMH difficulties.

---

10   www.tandfonline.com/doi/full/10.1080/02646838.2019.1649919

Mari: Yes! The thing with the census is that it has been a problem for a long time. I worked for the census the last time round. Before that I was working with data from the one before. I was working with the 2001 data in local government. Twenty years ago, we were saying it was difficult, and we just needed to ask the questions. I was out at that point, but it was the statistician in me that was calling for the data. Many of my cis het colleagues were also calling for the data, saying, 'Can we just ask the question please!' We were told we couldn't ask it because people wouldn't understand it, was too complicated and it was rude to ask. We seem to have now got to the point that we can include gender questions, but we still aren't asking about sexuality.

AJ: It's rude to ask the question, is it?

Mari: We have got another question in there now, which is: Do you identify with the gender you were assigned at birth? That question does need to be in there, of course it does. But where is the question about sexuality?

AJ: Given what we know about the breakdowns, even from the Stonewall documents and surveys, the disparities between the groups can be huge, so it's so important to get that data.

Mari: In maternity and perinatal services it's important because in correlating the free birth research, 4–5 per cent of the participants of the study were bisexual or lesbian women; 14 per cent of that group were planning a free birth.

AJ: Wow, that is a huge increase!

Mari: Huge! It is so significant. And it is the first time that it's been found – because it is the first time anyone has asked. My frustration is that we don't know what we are missing. We do know, for example from the MBBRACE[11] statistics, that black women are four to five times more likely to die in childbirth. Having that data alone doesn't mean we are doing enough about it or that having the data is what is important. But we don't even know if lesbians (or bisexual people assigned female at birth) are more likely to die.

I suspect that the answer is yes. I suspect that the answer is also yes for lesbians (and bisexual people assigned female at birth) being more likely to experience PMH difficulties. We just don't know because we are not asking the question. Even in the 20 years of my work, and campaigning for the question to be asked, it's still not being asked.

AJ: Wow, 20 years.

Mari: The reasons we are given for it not being asked are ludicrous as well – it would make the form too long, the IT system won't support it. All these kinds of barriers. Helen and Ash from BSUH have showed us what you can do, with *just* a paper form.

AJ: Yes, and I think Covid has shown us just how quickly boxes and questions can be added to forms and IT systems when it is perceived necessary for the protection of healthcare professionals and service users.

Mari: Yes.

AJ: Adding questions to capture data on sexuality and gender identity would protect service users and healthcare professionals but also allow them to know who they are caring for and what additional work they may have to undertake for this group or community to improve outcomes.

Mari: Yes, I agree.

---

11   www.npeu.ox.ac.uk/assets/downloads/mbrrace-uk/reports/perinatal-report-2020-twins/MBRRACE-UK_Twin_Pregnancies_Confidential_Enquiry.pdf

AJ: I am often asked why I think that midwives or obstetricians aren't asking these questions and the answer is, it's not them, it's not their fault, it is the systems and the procedures that need to ask the questions. I don't think healthcare providers go through all this training, all this debt, dedicating their lives to helping people, just to get up in the morning and be homophobic or transphobic if queer people come in. Well as a rule of thumb anyway; there will be some people who go out of their way to harm LGBT+ service users.

Mari: Yep, absolutely.

AJ: But they cannot provide the best care that I know they want to provide, if they are not supported by the powers that be and the computer systems, from the top down if you like, to capture this data. We can't do anything else until we are capturing this data.

Mari: Yes, even in terms of my own experience as a birth mum. All the forms want details of the 'partner'. Sometimes they want medical history, and sometimes they want to access social aspects like domestic violence and home life. If you don't ask the gender of someone's partner or their sexual orientation, you can't signpost them to the right services.

AJ: So, are we talking about the difference between capturing the partner's details and the other half of the baby's biology here?

Mari: Yes.

AJ: We know that there have been unnecessary referrals to obstetricians, for example off the back of the non-gestational parent's medical history. This boggles the mind really that it could happen. However, when we look at the forms, designed for cis het couples, that LGBT+ families must try and squash and shape their information into, we see why that happens.

Mari: Yes, and they are missing data and therefore referrals that should happen. By putting in the partner (who is not biologically linked) they are missing an opportunity to capture the data of the donor or the other biological link, if it is known.

AJ: Absolutely. They could be asking, in the case of when it is a donor conception, do you have any information about the other half of the baby's biology that might be relevant? In the UK, we have very limited information given by clinics, if indeed people have used clinics. Not everyone uses a clinic in the UK. We could have people getting their sperm from North America where you are given a hell of a lot more information about them, medical history, ethnicity, family medical histories and more.

Mari: Yes, and from the EU where you are given more information. Or, of course, using a friend or a known donor.

AJ: There could be relevant information that parents know that would help the healthcare professional give better care, and because it's not being asked, or there is no way to properly record that information, it is falling through the cracks.

Mari: Yes, that is exactly the problem.

AJ: Just to circle back to referrals for social and emotional reasons then. Thinking about domestic violence and the like. Do you think there are damaging assumptions within same-sex families specifically that mean that a lot of referrals or flags aren't being raised?

Mari: That isn't something I have researched but we do know that pregnancy is a time that triggers domestic violence. We also know that if domestic violence already exists it can get worse during pregnancy too. My experience as a doula is that midwives may make assumptions that domestic violence (DV) and coercive control (CC) aren't factors in same-sex relationships. In situations where we have a trans person giving birth with a male partner, a cis male partner, there is an assumption that it is not a consideration there.

AJ: So, relationships that are perceived as same-sex relationships?

Mari: Yeah, I guess it is relationships where 'power' is assumed to be equal? Then violence won't be an issue. I have personally had several clients where I have had concerns about the relationship regarding DV or CC. I have found it very hard to raise that with midwives and other healthcare professionals during the maternity or perinatal period, because there is just no knowledge that it could be a thing.

AJ: It comes back again, doesn't it, to the patriarchy?

Mari: Oh yes, of course.

AJ: If there are two opposing groups, male and female, one is more likely to be the 'victor' and one more likely to be abused or oppressed in some way. The patriarchal assumption of who is the oppressor and who is oppressed can oppress cis men as well.

Mari: I think it's about power, not so much physical dominance. I don't think the assumption of who is the oppressor would necessarily be changed by who is the physically larger of the couple for instance. DV and CC happen, overwhelmingly between cis men and cis women, more in this group than any other, I am sure. Is this about physical strength and sex, or is it about gender roles? Because if it is about gender or sex then yes you would expect to see much, much less of it in lesbian relationships. If it's about gender roles and one person is pregnant and the other one isn't, then you would expect to see it at the same rates.

AJ: That makes sense.

Mari: Given what we know about lack of support and visibility for the LGBT+ community, would we expect to see it more?

AJ: I don't know what the predisposing factors are for people to be one part of a DV situation, and even then you would have to break that down into abuser or abusee. The answer may lie somewhere in there.

Mari: We do know that DV and PMH have a relationship. If we are missing these links, then we can't act accordingly for those at risk.

AJ: So, these reasons, and I use that term very loosely, that healthcare professionals move away from capturing the data, and indeed that the powers that be decided the data doesn't need to be captured, could be preventing lifesaving interventions.

Mari: It's not just about asking for or recording the data. I have been in situations as a doula where I haven't done anything special in terms of data capture or asking questions. It's that there has been an openness in me to see what is in front of me.

AJ: This reason not to ask because it is offensive to assume someone's LGBT+-ness is a wider societal problem where LGBT+ is still seen as less than or wrong, so it's offensive to assume or even ask that someone is LGBT+. Of course, that also comes back to the patriarchy and gender roles.

Mari: Absolutely, of course.

AJ: What is it that you would say to a healthcare professional who is concerned about asking the question? As a birth worker, and as an LGBT+ and as a researcher, what would you say?

Mari: I think the push must come from the top down. It can't go bottom up. It needs to be recognized from NHS England that this data is required. For example, the data we capture on ethnicity is very flawed, the categories are problematic, the way it is interpreted is problematic. That work can happen, but it is not happening well enough or quick enough.

AJ: We saw this a bit with the update this year to the MBRRACE statistics that women of mixed ethnicity were put into a separate category, but if the ethnicity was unknown, or unasked, they were assumed white.

Mari: Yeah, it's hugely problematic. I think that asking questions or educating the healthcare professional comes at that stage. When the questions are there but they aren't perfect, it is the point to try and improve things, but we don't even have the questions yet to ask. It's not perfect, obviously, and it doesn't mean we can stop trying to create better questions for ethnicity capture, but for the LGBT+ data capture we can't be asking questions of the healthcare professional when we don't even have flawed questions yet.

AJ: So, there is no point someone reading this book and thinking they are going to start asking these questions because there is no way to record the answers?

Mari: Yep. I mean they ask the question. They are probably already asking the question – clumsily asking 'Is Dad around?' and getting the answer they weren't expecting that there is no dad. All those kinds of things, it's not that they don't know or aren't told that they are caring for LGBT+ in some instances. It is just that there is no way to properly record LGBT+ families so we can't go back and look at the data to identify trends or people who are at risk.

The push for change needs to come from the top down, so hopefully someone from NHS England will read the book and decide to start a campaign to capture the data.

AJ: I have had phone calls from NHS England and Healthwatch and those kinds of places asking me to solve their 'drop down box paradox' of how to capture data on healthcare accessibility for mental health referrals during the pandemic. I told them to leave the boxes blank so each person can fill in their own details of their identity.

Mari: Yep! It would be great to see the Royal College of Obstetricians and Gynaecologists and the National Medical Council lobbying for this data to be captured.

AJ: Is there anything else I haven't asked that you think is relevant or that you want healthcare professionals to know, either from your lived experience, professional experience as a doula or as a researcher?

Mari: The only other issue that is one of the huge gaps we found is that there is nothing about trans and non-binary partners. Say if there is a cis woman who is pregnant and her partner is a trans woman, or a non-binary person, there is nothing there. That reflects the dearth of literature on partners. We do know that partners can experience PMH difficulties as well. We do know some of the factors that make that more likely. There are a few papers out there that look at lesbian co-mothers, and that potentially they have a higher rate of PMH problems. There is one study, included in our review, which says that if the partner has the capability to be pregnant themselves, then they are more likely to experience birth as a traumatic event, even though they aren't the one giving birth.

AJ: So, either a same-sex couple, lesbian, bisexual, pansexual women, and those assigned female at birth or non-binary/trans masculine people?

Mari: Yes. So, the assumption that you have a cis man in front of you when you have a trans masculine or non-binary person will impact the likelihood of that person suffering PMH difficulties.

AJ: I wonder if the reverse is true as well then. Are we discounting the effects of dysmorphia or dysphoria for trans feminine partners as well?

Mari: Yes, we could be.

AJ: I have supported families where the mum is a trans woman and the birthing parent is non-binary. And the effect of the mum being left out of breast- or chest-feeding discussions and so on, as it was all directed to the birthing person, was quite profound for her. She very much felt that she was not given the same care and treatment that gestational mothers would have been given. So, the impact for her could have been very detrimental to her PMH as a non-gestational mother.

Mari: Very much so. The gap of information and knowledge for inducing lactation is huge. There is very little out there. Then when you add trans-ness into the equation for trans women there is even less available for them. Specialist induced lactation protocols are needed. You can't use the same ones that are used for cis women. We need to also consider how HRT goes through milk if they are on HRT. As far as I know, there is no research into it. I've only found one paper on it.

AJ: Was it this one [showing Mari the one included in the book]?

Mari: Yes, it's one woman's journey, and although useful and wonderful, it is not research.

AJ: Particularly when you consider that you may end up with a well-meaning healthcare professional who follows, for example, the Newman protocol with inducing lactation but that method may be contraindicated by medication that the trans woman may or may not be on.

Mari: And to go further than that, we must consider what medication we give to people who are trying to suppress lactation. We give birth control pills for the hormones that suppress lactation. There is no evidence base there for any of this.

AJ: Yes, there are huge gaps in research and knowledge in so many areas.

Mari: There is also the assumption that all trans masculine people will want a caesarean birth because they are dysphoric about their vaginas. Being trans should be a reason for a maternity request for birth, but we need to ensure we stop short of assuming or insisting that everyone will want or need it. If we find out, as I am expecting we will, that lesbians have a higher rate of perinatal mortality, and a higher rate of intervention, it is essential we don't make assumptions about care pathways. We need to stop short of over-medicalizing queer birth.

The other thing is the known or unknown donors. You cannot take known donor sperm into a fertility clinic in the UK. Well, you can, but one of the parents, the non-gestational parent, must sign their rights away. In our situation, because we were using a known donor, our friend, we had to write statements that my wife wasn't going to be a parent. I had to write one, she had to, he had to as well; it was horrific. With IVF, you have a higher chance when using fresh sperm than frozen sperm. So, if we had gone down the route of him donating to use it through the clinic it would be frozen, and we would have had less of a chance. However, if a heteronormative couple are going through IVF and use their sperm, they can have fresh sperm, and so have a higher likelihood of success. It's not just a quick sign on a form.

AJ: There have been instances of same-sex couples being encouraged to lie to get access to services like IVF. To lie that they have been trying for X amount of time, the such like. And, I get it a bit, because it is the healthcare professional trying to help the family get access to services that they want or need, but it shouldn't have to be this way. The parenthood journey shouldn't begin with having to lie or devalue yourself to get the treatment you want, to get the treatment you need.

Mari: Yep, that happens all the time. There is a PMH knock-on from all this as well. We talk about conversion disorder, where somebody doesn't feel like they are a proper parent. It's usually when someone has become a new birth mum and they don't make the transition to parenthood.

How much does having had to write down and sign your rights away, and declare you are not a parent before the baby is even conceived, affect this? You then also have to read your partner's statement that they don't consider you a parent, because that is what you have to do to get the treatment you want.

If lesbians have IVF and use one woman's eggs but the other woman gestates the baby, then the one whose egg it is has to sign away all the rights.

You cannot have lesbian surrogacy; this is illegal. Whoever is giving the egg is the donor. Not a parent. In cases of cis het people or a gay male couple using surrogacy, they don't have to sign away their rights, but when it is lesbians you must.

AJ: Wow.

Mari: Yeah... How much does that then affect your transition into parenthood and how much does that contribute to a knock-on effect for perinatal mental health? There is no research, so we can't prove that it impacts PMH. But there is good evidence around predisposing factors that do make it more likely to experience poor PMH outcomes and we can make an educated assumption that this will contribute.

AJ: Wow. It once again circles back to the fact that because LGBT+ folk can seldom fit into the boxes that currently exist within maternity and perinatal mental health, they are left at further risk. Or they try to squeeze through or are squeezed through by those services as a round peg in a square hole.

Mari: It's not just LGBT+ parents as well, that's the thing. One in ten young people in the UK are raised by someone they think is their father, and they aren't. Improvement to these systems will, as you said earlier, benefit more than just the LGBT+ service users.

AJ: There are cracks in the system, and you can never cover them all up, but when we know there are so many people falling into these holes, we need do something to save those families and improve those outcomes. We aren't even at the point of acknowledging that some of these gaps exist because we are not capturing the data!

Mari: Yep, I agree.

*

Talking with Mari always leaves me feeling in awe of their commitment to change as well as their lived experience. Dr Mari Greenfield continues to create many firsts and lead the way in research into LGBT+ disparities in perinatal mental health and maternity service. Her input has been ineffable, and I can't thank her enough.

CHAPTER 7

Lactation

There are several protocols for inducing lactation. Inducing lactation means 'jump starting' your milk production in the absence of a pregnancy. This process may be undertaken by non-gestational parents, such as adoptive parents, partners of gestational parents, and parents who didn't feed at birth and want to start some days, weeks or even months after the baby's birth. The information isn't specific for LGBT+ parents, or for non-binary or trans individuals assigned male at birth.

Prolactin is the hormone responsible for lactation, produced in the pituitary gland. Indeed, men, women and babies can experience this. It's not uncommon for newborn babies to excrete milk from their nipples due to the increased levels of oestrogen that can cross the placenta into the baby. It's never normally a cause for concern.

Many lactating parents have concerns around making enough milk to meet their baby's needs. This will almost certainly also be the case for any parent who is inducing lactation or re-lactating. Until they can see the signs that their baby is growing well and thriving on their milk, they may not be fully confident in the process. Having a newborn baby who seems to constantly want to go to the breast/chest may add to this uncertainty. Yet this is very likely exactly what the baby will want to do. It is normal, especially for newborn babies, to seek comfort in the breast/chest of a loving parent.

It is important to remember, for every breast-/chest-feeding relationship, that babies go to the breast or chest not just for nourishment. It may be due to hunger, thirst, a need for comfort, warmth, bonding time and interaction with their parent. We must remember always that babies experience the 'fourth trimester'.[1] Most mammals are born with developed gross motor skills – think about horses, which come out walking basically, although in a primitive Bambi-like fashion. When human infants are born, they are much more vulnerable than a lot of mammals and rely on their parents or caregivers for everything.

The fourth trimester can be explained as a period of adjustment for both parents and babies after the birth. Babies do not know that humans are living in houses, with baby monitors, cots and prams. From an evolutionary point of view, they think if you put them down a sabre-toothed cat is going to come into the cave and eat them, which explains why babies don't like being put down! However, sadly, we exist in a society, in the developed world, where we are obsessed with babies being 'good'. The neighbours or the old lady in the street will often ask, 'Are they good?', by which they normally mean, do they let you put them down so you can crack on with life? My favourite rebuttal was 'Yeah, they are great! They need me constantly and cry if I put them down – great evolutionary behaviours to have!' Mildred from two doors down didn't ask me that again. Most baby gadgets, those on the top ten lists of things to buy when expecting, are designed to help get the baby to let you put them down: the chairs, swings, hammocks, snugs and nests, the white noise machines, rockers, cribs, dummies, even a plug-in buggy treadmill-type thing that rocks the baby in their buggy as if it was being pushed outside for a stroll. Now I am not against these products, if they buy much-needed space from the stressed-out hell that can be new parenthood. However, I hold issue with a society that insists that bad babies are the ones that show completely normal, evolutionary behaviours and good ones are the ones that don't cry if they are left. So, the fourth trimester is evolutionary and, at times, painfully normal and beneficial for you and your baby. Those new parents checking in on this chapter to find out why their new baby won't be put down because they are inducing lactation can, I hope, be suitably reassured.

---

1   www.nct.org.uk/baby-toddler/emotional-and-social-development/what-fourth-trimester

Parents may want to induce lactation for a variety of reasons. To bond with their baby, lighten the load for their partner, and arguably most importantly for the immeasurable benefits that breastmilk provides for the child. It isn't easy, as any parent who has re-lactated will tell you. Add to this the added restrictions on medication needed and access to skilled, supportive, knowledgeable and LGBT+ competent birth workers, breastfeeding services, and supporters. Even if they can get in through the doors of these places despite lack of funding from local councils, they may wonder if they are welcome anyway.

On the other hand, some parents will not be sure whether they want to provide milk for their baby directly from their body. They may have a history of distrust or dislike of their body; they may have suffered trauma, which makes even the idea too difficult. They may have had reconstructive chest surgery which might impact on their ability to nurse. For many parents, these will be reasons to choose to offer milk via bottles from the start. For others, considering feeding their baby at the breast/chest may provide an opportunity for healing past trauma. Any individual may not know what will suit them best until they are expecting a baby, or even after their baby is born. It may help to find someone to speak to whom they trust to help work out what is the right path for them.

Any parent may be able to induce lactation. The likelihood of that parent being able to obtain their feeding goals may hinge on the support they receive from healthcare professionals, lay persons and loved ones.

Support and knowledge for non-gestational parents' breast- or chest-feeding is very sparse in general. However, for trans women who want to breast-/chest-feed, there is even less out there for them.

Reisman and Goldstein (2018) published an article in the journal *Transgender Health* about a case of induced lactation: 'Case report: Induced lactation in a transgender woman'.[2] It details the case of a 30-year-old transgender woman who provided enough milk to exclusively breastfeed her baby for six weeks. The report details the

---

2   www.liebertpub.com/doi/10.1089/trgh.2017.0044

hormones she had taken in the years prior to the baby's birth, and changes made to her hormone supplements to induce lactation. In addition, she took a known galactagogue (domperidone) and stimulated milk production by pumping the breasts with a breast pump. Her partner, the gestational parent, did not intend to breastfeed. Following the schedule detailed in the article, which is available online, the woman produced enough milk to breastfeed her baby exclusively for six weeks, and then continued to breastfeed alongside some supplementation with formula up until publication of the article, at which time the baby was still being mixed fed at the age of six months.

What this article proves is that it is possible for trans women to lactate. What percentage of the milk her baby needs she can make will be dependent on many things. The physiological and psychological benefits of breastfeeding are not lost or to be discarded based on the volume of human milk.

The physiological impact for parent and child also cannot be diminished based on quantity or percentages of total milk produced.

Partners of gestational parents may also need support with inducing lactation. This may be a lesbian couple, or a dyad of two or more persons assigned female at birth, or indeed male at birth. Those who are assigned female at birth will have a biological 'advantage' over their assigned male at birth cohort.

We will meet a couple in our real-life examples later, who experienced difficulty in the non-gestational mother gaining access to the postnatal ward to allow the baby to go to the breast. With all the protocols and suggestions in ways to increase the likelihood that lactation is successful, it is stated that the baby should be encouraged to go to the breast as much as possible, and have as much skin-to-skin contact with the parent inducing lactation as possible.

Skin-to-skin is very simple and free, holding the baby with their skin against yours. It's been used for centuries to calm babies and indeed its use in what we in modern terms call 'kangaroo care' has seen remarkable results. UNICEF (United Nations Children's Emergency Fund) tells us that having skin-to-skin contact with a baby can regulate the baby's and parent's heart rate and temperature, stimulate their interest in feeding and increase oxytocin for the parent (another hormone which is essential in breast milk production and general parenting).[3] Restricting access to those who aren't the gestational mother but are wishing to induce lactation puts another barrier in the way of families and their breast-/chest-feeding goals. Yes, hospitals will have their policies, but hospitals and birthing centres exist to make us better, to aid us. So, if you work in a hospital, why not ask about the policy for non-gestational parents having access to the postnatal ward when they need to see their baby for the purposes of re-lactation? Then, when a teary-eyed parent comes to you needing to be with their baby, you will already have the knowledge and have started the conversation within your NHS trust about the procedure. If you are an expectant parent, this may be a good question to add to the list you have for your healthcare provider. Even if you are having a home birth or attending a standalone birthing centre, it may be useful to know this information ahead of time in case of transfer to hospital.

Additionally, what are the business/trust's guidelines for families who have used a surrogate to grow their families? Are all the intended parents allowed in the postnatal ward? Is it limited to just one parent?

It is a balancing act to ensure that the breastmilk supply of the gestational parent is guarded if they are choosing to breastfeed or continue to breastfeed themselves. Sharing out the skin-to-skin time and putting the baby to the breast will be tricky. No parent wants to suffer with mastitis (an infection caused by breastmilk being insufficiently drained from the breast). Gestational/non-gestational parents should be mindful that whoever will be the baby's 'main' milk supplier, for want of a better term, should take precedence in the pecking order to ensure that the supply of breastmilk is guaranteed.

Some non-gestational parents may want the baby to take to the breast just for comfort. I have indeed seen a cis hetero man nurse their newly born baby while the mum was being attended to by midwives.

---

3   www.unicef.org.uk/babyfriendly/baby-friendly-resources/implementing-standards-resources/skin-to-skin-contact

Non-gestational parents, men and women, have a long history of 'comfort suckling' their babies. Including aunts, uncles and other loved ones of the baby, we were doing this well before there were midwives, doctors and hospitals. It is normal and biological. Dummies are a replacement breast/chest, so don't forget that when someone will inevitably say that the baby is using you 'as a dummy'. Knowing what we do about the fourth trimester, we would all be mindful to remember that babies don't 'just' use a nipple for comfort – it is so, so much more than that.

Some parents inducing lactation may find using a supplemental nursing system (SNS) effective. This is a thin tube attached to a milk source – this could be a syringe or a bottle – that is then placed at the nipple of the parent, and as the baby latches, they latch on to the tube and the nipple at the same time. The milk then flows from the milk receptacle and, it is hoped, the parent. Many parents use this method, whether they are inducing lactation or not. They may be encouraging weight gain in a slight baby, or trying to increase breastmilk supply, or trying to get over bottle preference (a baby may develop a bottle preference when some or all the milk is offered in a bottle and it is easier for the baby to remove larger amounts of milk faster from an artificial teat than the chest/breast).

Trevor MacDonald, in his book,[4] talks at length about the practicalities and difficulties in using an SNS for 'top ups' of donor milk while feeding his baby. An SNS can be used for both donor milk and infant formula milk. Trevor's book is a treasure trove of information and essential for anyone who wants to work with all manner of folk, particularly those who have had top surgery.

In any cases where breast-/chest-feeding advice is needed, it's best that it comes from someone qualified and experienced in breastfeeding.

In the UK, we have the International Board of Certified Lactation Consultants (IBCLCs), which offers the highest and most renowned qualification that a person can get in breastfeeding, requiring a

---

4   MacDonald, T. (2016) *Where's the Mother?* Manitoba: Trans Canada Press

staggering 1000 hours of face-to-face support in breastfeeding to even get on to the course. Sadly, people with this qualification are often only available privately due to lack of funding in our NHS. Some trusts are lucky to have them on their rotas. Some who work privately may offer reduced or no cost support through Pay It Forward schemes or via drop-ins. It is worth looking into what is available in your area. If funds are a barrier, you may also find someone who has a Pay It Forward scheme and is able to offer support via video, even if they are not in your local area. Many consultants have developed their skills in video support because of restrictions during the Covid-19 pandemic. Some will continue to work online, which will also allow parents to find professionals who can work with them in a safe and inclusive way, even if they do not live nearby.

When checking out hospitals or postnatal services in their local area, new or prospective parents may also want to find out who the infant feeding team are, how they can be reached on the phone and in person, along with what children centres, if any, have breastfeeding drop-ins, and who there might provide support. Is there a La Leche League[5] meeting nearby, or another breastfeeding meet-up?

Unfortunately, GPs receive little to no training in breastfeeding and lactation, and other well-meaning healthcare professionals may not be able to adequately help either, unless they have undertaken additional training in lactation.

We also have the National Breastfeeding Helpline, staffed by qualified and experienced breastfeeding counsellors from the Association of Breastfeeding Mothers, and the Breastfeeding Network. Volunteers will be happy to speak to you on the phone, and/or refer you to face-to-face groups:

National Breastfeeding Helpline: 0300 100 0212, 9.30am–9.30pm
National Childbirth Trust (NCT): 0300 330 0700, 8am–midnight
La Leche League: 0345 120 2918, 8am–11pm

---

5   La Leche League is a breastfeeding support network.

CHAPTER 8

We Actually Exist

It seems to be too easy for people to say, 'There just isn't an LGBT+ population in my area so I don't need to consider or be aware of the issues you are talking about.' Let me tell you, we exist, we are out there. You have probably shared space with us on public transport, in restaurants and toilets already. You cannot always tell, you cannot always see us for looking. That sometimes gives us protection and safety and sometimes it is crushing to be invalidated or erased because we don't walk, talk, act, dress or seem 'gay' to you.

Some of the following stories were shared with me by Dr Mari Greenfield, a lesbian birth and foster parent who has been a doula for over a decade, and midwife Nathan Welch. Some were told to me by the parents directly.

The stories were gleaned by Mari and Nathan through various channels, from presentations, research and from Mari's own doula work. All people in the examples have given their permission for them to be used. The headings have been lifted directly from Mari and Nathan's work, with their permission, and I have gone on to discuss and explain the issues further.

They aren't there to serve as catch-all examples of ways services are currently lacking in their provisions and awareness of those who birth outside the cis heteronormative world. They are simply the real-life, real-deal experiences of people who have navigated the systems. They will serve a purpose and I thank those involved very much for allowing their stories to be shared.

When looking at these examples, ask yourself a few questions along the way:

- Would this happen in my NHS trust or business? Are the current systems that we use going to have the same holes or pitfalls that parents in a similar situation could fall through or into?
- What could be done, if anything, to ensure that parents in a similar situation wouldn't experience these same disparities?
- Could I highlight this example to my superiors or policy changers?
- Would I know how to advocate or speak to these parents? Am I, unconsciously or consciously, contributing to these restrictions, disparities, biases and assumptions?

Asking yourself these questions can be difficult. It can bring up feelings of guilt or worry that parents are experiencing this in your NHS trust. Take care of yourself as you work through these pages.

What you choose to do about those feelings is up to you. It is hoped that these feelings will be used as motivation for real change. All the examples are from the UK, and some names have been changed to protect the identity of those involved.

Case studies

Katherine and Vicky

- They have one child already (Katherine gave birth).
- Donor insemination at home was unsuccessful for a second baby, to be carried by Vicky.
- Wished to have fertility treatment using their donor, so that the children would be biologically half-siblings.
- Fertility clinics have an ethical responsibility for the health of the baby. Therefore, there is no access to fertility treatment with a known donor and they have to use a donor from the

clinic, which means that their children will not be biologically related.

Although on the surface this seems rather self-explanatory, it's rather complex when you consider the legal implications of accessing known and unknown donors.

As previously discussed in Chapter 5, How Did You Even Get Pregnant Anyway?, you cannot use a known or private donor in fertility clinics. (Well, you might be able to, but you may have to sign your rights away, as Dr Greenfield told us in Chapter 6.) There are many reasons for this, but the most common is that they cannot guarantee the health of the baby or the specimen (sperm in this instance but can also mean eggs) without the donor and their specimen(s) going through screening (for conditions such as HIV, hepatitis etc.).

There may also then be legal repercussions as to who is the father or co-parent of the baby. When a specimen is provided through a clinic, parental rights are waived, and therefore when the baby is born there is an 'automatic' parental right to the baby if the couple are in a civil partnership or married. This is difficult when you are not then the father, as defined by law as the 'biological father, who impregnated the mother'. So again, we see it's a very complicated matter, and assuming that your clients are this far along in the process it is likely that they are aware of their rights and the process; however, most families using home insemination will likely take legal counsel, to ensure that everyone is clear and signed on the dotted line for their responsibilities and roles in the child's life, if any at all.

This leaves Katherine and Vicky in a situation where they have to use an unknown donor at a clinic in order to access the help they needed, but their children will not be biologically related as per their wishes.

Do you know the processes at your local fertility clinic? Having an even small base of knowledge on the subject would go a long way to fostering a positive and trusting relationship with clients who use donation to grow their families.

Ian and Mark

- Ian is pregnant with his and Mark's third genetic child. Testing revealed Anti-Kell antibodies.
- Time to treatment is of the essence with Anti-Kell.
- There are ten attempts to have maternal blood tests for Ian – but paternal tests are carried out each time 'because he's a man'.
- Then first paternal blood test on Mark shows no problem (not medically possible).
- NHS insists a previous child must not be Mark's, or Ian must be a medical miracle.
- Subject access request shows that the wrong test has been conducted on Mark too – a maternal one has been used.

This is a heart-breaking but fantastic example of how we cannot fit into the boxes on forms and what effect this can have on trans and non-binary parents. It can and has put lives at risk.

Anti-Kell or haemolytic disease is a condition in which the antibodies in a pregnant person's blood cross the placenta and destroy the baby's red blood cells, causing severe anaemia. This condition results when there is a mismatch between the parent's and the baby's blood group Kell antigens. If careful monitoring of the baby isn't carried out, or it is missed at the standard blood test offered to all pregnant people in the UK at around 17–20 weeks, then there is a real risk of the baby being born with severe life-limiting or life-ending conditions of the heart and lungs.

When carrying out the blood tests on Ian they have sent his blood for the specific testing done for 'fathers' as Ian is a man. It shows that there is no cause for concern because they have done the wrong tests. Later they find out that the hospital has also done maternal tests on Mark's blood; clearly it was all too confusing, so they just sent the lot for every test.

It is important to confirm the other half of the baby's DNA when discussing Anti-Kell, but insisting that Mark cannot be the father could be enough to break some relationships. Also consider the impact on these words if either parent is abusive, emotionally or physically. Insisting that a parent is not the biological parent could have a catastrophic impact on the mental health of those parents, and give fuel to a fire of abuse.

In this example, it has happened because of an inability or unwillingness to record a patient's relationship to their baby in a way that is biologically accurate and true to Ian and Mark.

Would having an open and frank conversation with Ian and Mark to explain that because of the way the system/forms/process works we have to mark down 'woman' or 'mother' on these test requests and apologizing (and trying to fix that process if it is possible, of course!) have prevented this from happening?

Would having an extra box on form requests to explain any 'unusual' situations have been useful for the phlebotomist? In both options, having the vocabulary and bedside manner to execute these discussions is essential and emphasizes the need for an understanding of terminology to competently care for LGBT+ parents.

Some of the midwives I have spoken to in workshops about this example have asked whether a transgender person acquiring a GRC (gender recognition certificate – the legal document required to change gender markers on official documents or certificates) changes their NHS number. The answer is yes, when a GRC is issued a new NHS number is generated. All the history of that patient therefore could be difficult to obtain. Imagine having to work with all your service users with no or limited history? As this is now something you are aware of, how will that change how you care for trans folk who have a GRC?

This could have ended in a very different manner, but I am happy to report that Ian and Mark had a happy and healthy baby, once they got the healthcare professional to realize what on earth was going on here, and how they even got pregnant in the first place.

Mary and Jameelah

- Mary is pregnant.

- Their midwife wants to be inclusive, so on the maternity notes crosses out 'father', and inserts 'partner'.
- The midwife then records Jameelah's details in the space for 'father'.
- The maternity system makes a referral to a neonatal consultant, based on Jameelah's family's medical history.

This story is opposite in a way to Ian and Mark's story. It is interesting to consider that on top of the unnecessary referral to neonatal consultant, wasting time, money and worry for parents and the NHS, we are also left wondering what could have been missed in this well-intentioned but wild stab at inclusion. If Mary and Jameelah had used a known donor they may have been aware or unaware of the donor's history that needed to be recorded or might be a reason for referral.

It is good to want to be inclusive but doing so with little awareness of how this could affect your clients or patients' access to healthcare or limit their choices is dangerous, as Mary and Jameelah's story demonstrates.

Knowing that conditions or history of the non-gestational parent could be cause for referral or additional tests, which may carry their own risks, healthcare professionals must understand the balance between due diligence and meaningful history taking.

Some NHS trusts have forms that have a tick box or a separate box for parents who are not the other half of the baby's biology, thinking about those who conceive their babies using IVF as well. What is the process in your trust or service?

A midwife who attended one of my workshops was successful in implementing an 'additional information' box on the top of her notes. Even a sticker may be possible, to highlight to all those taking care of this family that there are special considerations. Some trusts already use these stickers for parents who have experienced miscarriage or stillbirth, to alert them to medical history that could help them provide better, more personalized care for those families who choose to use their services.

In this example, I do feel for the midwife. I see so clearly that her thought process was to be inclusive and give Jameelah the standing that she deserves on these documents. However, it is a powerful and timely reminder that *your intent does not negate your impact*. How you think your actions will be received or how you think your actions will change the care that this family receives don't always add up. It's great to have fabulous inclusive motives, but being able to look forward and predict how these changes could impact these service users is an act of allyship.

It is important that Jameelah's name is on these documents, in her rightful place of non-gestational parent. Consider the legal implications of parentage if anything were to happen to Mary. Who will care for this child? Who has the right to make decisions about care or treatment? As we discussed previously, this can be complicated. Knowing if Mary and Jameelah are married or in a civil partnership will mean whether or not Jameelah, as the non-gestational parent, will have to apply for adoption for her baby. If they are married, then Jameelah will be recorded as parent two on the baby's birth certificate, but what does this mean in the interim between the baby's birth and the baby being issued with a birth certificate?

The government website tells us that a mother has automatic parental responsibility for her child from birth. It also tells us that the father usually has parental responsibility if he's either married to the child's mother or listed on the birth certificate. Civil partners in same-sex relationships will both have parental responsibility if they were civil partners at the time of the treatment (e.g. donor insemination or fertility treatment). For non-civil partners, the second parent can obtain parental responsibility by either applying for it if a parental agreement was made or becoming the civil partner of the other parent and making a parental responsibility agreement or jointly registering the birth.

The current process does leave unmarried non-gestational parents in a strange limbo during the period of birth and registration of the baby. Knowing the parent's situation before birth, particularly if the baby is expected to need some medical treatment after birth, will be an act of allyship for those parents and their baby. Again, this relies on being aware of the legalities and having the language to ask the questions in a manner that doesn't alienate or destroy trust between care provider and service user.

Jay

- Jay is a single, pregnant, non-binary person, who takes testosterone and has a masculine appearance.
- Induction of labour is indicated.
- The hospital they have planned to give birth in has no single rooms for induction, only six-bed wards.
- At the second hospital, admission is cancelled twice when Jay arrives, as the single rooms are already in use.
- The induction of their labour is delayed by a week due to these problems.

This example really speaks for itself. We don't know whether the private room was at the request of the hospital or Jay themselves, but having an induction delayed based on housekeeping would impact on anyone's birth.

As we know already, not being able to relax, feel safe, cared for and loved is not conducive to birth and the cocktail of hormones that needs to happen, even during an induction.

Inductions are often cancelled or delayed at the last minute due to demand on maternity units. I have supported families where they have been told to go on Friday at 8am only to be turned away when they arrive as instructed as the unit is full or too busy. They are often told to come back on Monday or another date, which, considering induction or augmentation of labour is meant to be reserved for medical necessity rather than bed or room availability, is incredibly cruel for parents to be. They are thrust into this never-neverland of waiting for their induction when they should be focusing on the life-changing process which is about to unfold for them.

Some trusts operate on a system of private rooms for pay, or private rooms being available for those with medical need. Given the risk for LGBT+ people out in the wider world, surely it would be wise to offer private rooms or facilities for LGBT+ parents. The key word here being offer. Some parents may appreciate the offer and feel safer with some privacy. I have supported families, particularly trans masculine parents, who feel wracked with guilt that their presence in a labour ward will make other service users fearful. Also there are some service users who have a religious necessity to be in a space without men. I have also worked with parents who were excited to be in the open labour ward to share this experience with other parents and be able to socialize with other brand-new parents.

The choice should be that of the parents themselves; however, if the next family to walk into your service is trans and asks if you are able to give them a private room on the basis that their gender identity puts them at risk, do you know what your trust's policy is on that? Asking the hard questions before an LGBT+ person must is an act of allyship.

Pelagia and Renee

- Lesbian couple, having their first baby.
- During labour, a new midwife comes into the room, and asks, 'So, how did *this* happen?'
- This is the story they still recall about the birth, 15 years later.

The last sentence is the one that sticks with me, knowing how much parents need to and want to talk about their birth, and to have this moment marred on their journey makes my heart ache.

It does, however, illustrate my earlier point of asking questions to satisfy your own curiosity rather than out of medical necessity or, in Mary and Jameelah's case, to be 'inclusive'.

Having a healthcare professional, to whom you are meant to entrust the most vulnerable but powerful moments of your life, more interested in how you got pregnant than how you are doing, how they can help you, is destroying. We are not sideshows or purely educational or diversity subjects, we are real people, birthing our real babies, and we need love and validation as much as the next cis, straight couple coming through the doors.

I doubt that it was the intention of the midwife to hurt Pelagia and Renee. It may have been, but it is more likely, in my opinion and experience, that this was simply a poorly executed stab for information. Again, we must come back to the point that having the language and terminology to ask questions about service users and their journey to pregnancy is an essential part of being competent when caring for LGBT+ parents. It's also vital to know the difference between when it is essential to ask these questions and asking purely for your own curiosity. Was this question, however badly or brilliantly worded, necessary? At this very moment? Was it essential? There may very well be times where you need to ask questions about biology, about the baby's parentage, history and so on, but remember to first ask yourself why you are asking.

Ian and Mark

- First birth in hospital.
- On arrival in labour at the labour ward, access is via an intercom.
- Between contractions, they try to explain who they are.
- They are denied access to the labour ward 'until the mum arrives'.

We meet Ian and Mark again for another example of how trans and non-binary bodies are treated differently in and around the birth and baby world.

During contractions, Mark and Ian try to explain why they need to come in, in what we can probably assume is an open and possibly busy hospital corridor.

Fighting your way into a maternity unit isn't what any parent needs when they are starting their journey into parenthood. On top of being repeatedly denied the possibility of their existence and the ability to birth their baby before they have even entered the doors no doubt has a biological, chemical effect on both Ian and Mark, activating their fight or flight or adrenaline when they should have been allowed to focus on their then and now.

Most hospitals have intercoms now. The safety of everyone on the ward is paramount, and we understand why, of course, access to places where some of the most vulnerable members of our society are is guarded and protected.

During workshops, a lot of doulas and midwives often ask why the person on the other end wasn't aware that the arrival of a man in labour was expected or imminent.

I have seen in labour ward handovers complex or unusual cases being discussed so that everyone is aware of who may be coming in. I have supported parents who wanted a vaginal birth after caesarean or had a vaginal breech birth and they were the hot topic of conversation at handovers so that everyone was aware that maybe during the shift they would need attention.

I am not suggesting for one minute that all LGBT+ parents should be announced with a fanfare onto maternity wards or birthing units up and down the country. However, the midwife or admin member of staff who was working that evening being aware that at some point a man is going to come in may have prevented the situation for Ian and Mark.

Another solution that people often offer is that the member of staff at the other end of the intercom could have simply gone and spoken to the family face to face. This might not always be possible, but it is another option. Ian and Mark may have called ahead to let the unit know that they were inbound. This isn't always the case, and, in some situations, they may have just turned up, but it is another argument for one-to-one care. Having someone meet them at the hospital entrance, for example, may have been another solution.

Making assumptions about what people will look like and who needs access to our service can have a catastrophic impact on the service user's experience and safety. The person on the other end of the intercom knowing that trans men can, and do, give birth and need access to maternity units may have also prevented Ian and Mark starting their experience of becoming parents in hospital on such a footing.

Branwen and Ffion

- Branwen is pregnant.
- Ffion is intending to fully breastfeed, and has followed a lactation protocol.
- They knew before the birth that their baby would need to spend a few days in hospital afterwards.
- But Ffion is only allowed in during visiting hours. They complain about this.
- The NHS reply to their complaint upholds the policy, and states that 'fathers are not allowed on the ward overnight'.

When non-birthing parents (including adoptive parents) want to breastfeed, they may be able to induce lactation. This requires a lot of work for both parents. If the birthing parent is also planning to breastfeed then they will also need access to the baby. The parent trying to induce lactation requires as much skin-to-skin time as possible, as well as having the baby go to the breast/chest.

Having a blanket policy that restricts parents' access to babies will inevitably create instances where parents feel unsupported and are alienated. In cases like this, it could mean that inducing lactation is extremely difficult or even impossible.

Some NHS trusts allow you to have your partner with you at any time; other trusts allow them to stay the first night, and some allow no access outside normal visiting hours, so it's worth checking with the hospital to ensure that the staff can be made aware of the needs of the families.

The use of language in the response to Branwen and Ffion's complaint is another example of how we don't fit into the boxes and standard responses, and how we can fall through the cracks in policies and procedures.

It's also worth considering the rights of the baby – their right to be fed and cared for by their parents. I have heard of some NHS trusts wanting to restrict visiting to just those with parental rights. Again, thinking back to the discussion on parental rights with same-sex couples, or unmarried couples in general, this may be excluding whole groups of biological, non-biological or intended parents from having access to their babies, as well as being able to support their loved one during this vulnerable time.

It also begs questions about any accreditation that hospitals may have or be working towards like BFI (Baby-Friendly Initiative).

With all families, it is common to make assumptions about who will feed the baby, and how. Young parents are often assumed to be bottle-feeding parents and older parents are assumed to be more likely to breast- or chest-feed their babies. A lot of same-sex couples that I speak to don't even know it is possible for the non-gestational parent to breast-/chest-feed the baby. I don't know many parents who wouldn't have given a lot of money to be able to hand the baby to someone else in those never-ending cluster feeds or burnt-out, stressed moments. Making parents aware that this is an option, and that there are services that exist to help them in their journey, is an act of allyship.

Ellie and Louie

- Ellie is a cis woman and Louie is a trans man.
- When they want to access fertility treatment, they are told that the centre will have to decide whether to treat them as a same-sex couple or a heterosexual couple.
- Their NHS trust won't fund fertility treatment for same-sex couples using sperm donation, but they will cover a heterosexual couple as it would be considered a fertility issue.
- The trust decides to treat Ellie and Louie as a heterosexual couple and therefore they qualify for NHS funding.
- However, because the 'pathway for funding' means an investigation into the fertility issue between the couple, Ellie has

to have several procedures, including a keyhole surgery under general anaesthetic.

The sheer lack of common sense in this one always upsets and baffles me!

How can we subject women and birthing people to unnecessary risk purely because of the pathway they are on, which makes it necessary to have these procedures?

It is worth pointing out that the fertility issue here is that Ellie and Louie don't have any sperm. There is no proof that there is an issue. But, for them to proceed with the NHS fertility service, they are required to explore why they can't get pregnant. When one of the essential components isn't available, it seems cruel at best and negligent at worst to subject them to these risks.

It again highlights that this system is set up expecting cisgender heterosexual clients. Therefore, when a family doesn't fit that narrow expectation, they are not only at increased risk from the outside world, but also at risk from the healthcare systems.

During this whole process, it is astounding to me that no one once said 'Oh wait, I know what the issue is!' and was able to bypass the computer system or the referral system for this family to get the help that they need and deserve.

Postcode lotteries for access to treatment are very common in the NHS and affect everyone, not just LGBT+ parents, although there is a need for a pathway for LGBT+ parents.

All this is upsetting. All of it stems from a world and a system centred around cis and heterosexual parents.

If we want to end these disparities for LGBT+ parents, then we need to be asking questions. Who is left behind using this system? Who isn't being considered here? Who can't be recorded accurately? Why aren't there any LGBT+ parents/people on this panel? Why are these focus groups just focusing on mums or birthing parents? Why isn't there a procedure in place to bypass this system when we have a same-sex or LGBT+ family?

Asking these questions now before an LGBT+ family has to is an essential act of allyship.

Fran and George

- Fran is non-binary and pregnant, and George is their cis male bisexual partner.
- They hire a doula for the birth of their second child.
- Everything goes well and they have an incredible, healing birth at home without medical intervention just as they had hoped.
- Some time later the doula posts transphobic rhetoric on her social media declaring that all who birth are women and female.
- Comment from Fran: 'My identity being erased was one thing, but now, when I think of my birth, I think of whose hand I was holding rather than my achievements, or even my baby.'

Whenever I talk about this example during workshops, it elicits anger and disbelief. Fran's words at the end are a heart-breaking but monumentally telling part of the story.

The reason I include this example is to get people to think about the impact of their words, especially in an ever-growing digital age. We never know who is looking at what we write, or who is listening to what we say. It also reminds us that unless we ask, we do not know the gender identity of the people we are caring for. The doula here could have assumed that they were a cisgender heterosexual couple and may not have even known that she was caring for a trans person. She may have known and taken the job anyway, for many reasons. This is a reminder that you cannot see gender or pronouns. Unless you ask, you could be doing a tremendous disservice to your service users, and contributing to a negative outcome, emotionally or physically.

This example also makes us consider what we would do if someone in our NHS trust, our community, someone who worked under the same umbrella as us, did something comparable. Maybe it would be someone who trained on the same doula course. How would you react?

What actions would you take if a colleague made trans exclusionary or homophobic statements on social media or in the wider world?

There are plenty of people around with these opinions. They are often loudly and strangely proud of their opinion that trans people don't exist or are not deserving of inclusion in matters of maternity/paternity.

Often it is thought that allyship must be just as loud or just as aggressive as the voices who harm us, that the fact that LGBT+ can be parents is an argument to be won. There aren't two valid sides to this argument. There are facts. LGBT+ parents are just as deserving to access services and the love and care of healthcare professionals and lay persons as their non-LGBT+ cohort. The rest is just noise. It isn't anyone's job to convince with statistics or figures that this is true or valid. It is up to the allies to stand by the LGBT+ community to ensure that those whose loud shouts of erasure and violence aren't held higher or equal to the voices of the oppressed.

How would you plan to counter these voices?

Archbishop Desmond Tutu said that 'if you are neutral in situations of injustice, you have chosen the side of the oppressor'. Therefore, if someone in your circle, class, trust, group, space states that trans people don't need rights in maternity, or that by including the language or imagery of LGBT+ families it is somehow taking away from the cis or the hetero, and no objection is heard, the lack of objection gives space and time to the oppressor's words or actions. Silence by proxy agrees. The recourse to words doesn't have to be as loud, or as violent, but only you can decide if or how to challenge these views.

Within this conversation we must acknowledge that it is not always safe to show allyship. If you are at risk yourself if you were to, for example, be the lone voice in objection and you fear for your safety through repercussions, don't put yourself in harm's way.

Mounting your objection could take the form of sharing some LGBT+ content on a day where LGBT+ parents are under attack. It could be posting a book, channel or workshop recommendation. It could be donating to a charity that supports the community that is under attack. It could be silent and quiet work on your own bias or assumptions. Allyship has many forms.

Jenny and Samantha

- Jenny is labouring in a hospital.
- The midwife says: 'I don't get it. Why you do have to "push it in my face"?'
- Samantha asks what the midwife means.
- The midwife continues by asking why they must push their sexuality in her face by holding hands and so on.
- A complaint is filed, pending investigation and outcome.

This example was given to me the day before I was due to travel to the university attached to this very hospital to give a workshop to the student midwives there. I like to include this example for the workshops I do online because, unfortunately, it shows that, pure and simple, homophobia does exist within individuals.

It is important to ask yourself what you would do if a member of your team or organization behaved in this way. Even more awkwardly, you must ask yourself if you think this way. Have you, unconsciously or consciously, over-sexualized LGBT+ people to the point where everything they do, including physically comforting their loved one during labour, is viewed as sexualized or as weaponized sexuality?

When people hear this example, some insist that homophobic midwives should make themselves known and be barred from caring for LGBT+ service users. I have also had opinions that the midwife herself should have declined to care for this family, removing herself from the equation. This relies on the midwife being aware that these are biases or 'phobias' that she has. It also relies on the LGBT+ parents being treated differently. It also brings up whether LGBT+ midwives should always be the ones to care for LGBT+ parents. Some LGBT+ midwives express frustration at always being given or asked if they could support the LGBT+ service users, based purely on the shared experience of their LGBT+ identities. Although on the surface this may seem like common sense to have people that look like you, think like you or walk through the world like you to care for you, it should never be dictated or expected. All healthcare professionals should be adequately trained, supported and proud to be able to serve, support and love all those who need their services. If being able to properly support and care for people who need your service depends on them fulfilling certain criteria such as who they love, where they are from, what language they speak, what religion they are or what the colour of their skin is, then there are bigger factors at play here than access to services.

Interviews

Kayden Coleman: Seahorse Papa

I have followed Kayden for a long time now. I get so much from his account, and I bet you will too. Kayden himself, his courses, his social media account are so important. He seldom pulls back or stifles his voice, and he shouldn't. He speaks about allyship and intersectionality so powerfully, I knew he was the man to tell us about allyship.

> The biggest part of allyship is being willing to learn, and to unlearn the biases and assumptions you have made; to constantly and continually be learning.
>
> The best experience of allyship I can think of is having someone in the medical field who knew who I was. They didn't treat me like an anomaly. She wasn't a doctor or a midwife, she was a receptionist. When I found out I was pregnant with my second child, I called in to the centre, because I had heard they were trans competent. I purposefully didn't say I was trans at the start of the call, I said, 'I am pregnant, I just found out, I just did a test', and the first thing she said was, 'Okay, that's great, I have a question for you. Are you trans?' I was so taken aback and happy. She didn't ask me if I was calling for my wife or my friend, she didn't say, 'Sir, you have the wrong number!', or anything like that. When I went in, she made sure to schedule me on days when she was there so

she would be the person to check me in and give me the forms and so on. If there was a time when she wasn't there, she did a really great job of letting people know the deal and who to expect to come in. If there was a referral to another clinic or service, she would call ahead, with me there beside her to let them know that, yes, he is coming in, he is pregnant, these are his pronouns and so on. She stood by me.

Another situation was after I gave birth to my second daughter. The nurse was standing there chatting with the doctor about my care needs and all that, and she kept misgendering me. You could tell it was making the doctor uncomfortable too because he was shifting and looking over at me. He just spoke over her and said, 'He! You mean he.' She was just quite taken aback and started to try to explain away what she was doing, 'Well you have to understand this is difficult for me', but he didn't entertain that for a second. He said, 'No, it's part of your job to support people correctly, use he.' To have those kinds of people standing up for you in that very vulnerable situation was priceless really. When it comes to trans-ness as a whole, in the medical community, if I am getting misgendered and call this out, it will make the situation worse or more uncomfortable. How do I go about letting them know that this is not okay without causing this friction? We're in this vulnerable state, because our health is literally in their hands. When you are in a position that women are typically in as well, it's kind of hard to judge how they will react to being called out. Maybe that hasn't happened before.

Those two examples stand out to me more than all the shit because they were so refreshing.

For anyone who wants to be an ally, the best way is to show up. Educate yourself, attend trans-led trainings and workshops and Facebook events, instead of trying to get the information from a cis person. We see it all the time, cis people running these courses. I did see a birth worker doing this and she was honest and said from the start I can't sit here and tell you all of this because I don't know. I am not a member of this community. This is just the bare bones, what does trans mean, all this basic stuff. I can't tell you what I don't know. Her son is trans, so she does have some personal connection with the trans community, but she didn't try to sell it as if it was her experience.

The other important aspect is to be continuously learning. What I mean is that you can't do one course run by someone in 2010 and then expect to be able to keep up with everyone's needs and wants in (the present).

Also important to me is not just taking advice from a certain type of trans person. What I mean is, you have white, het birth workers or pregnant people and everyone flocks to them because it's more palatable for them. I tell people all the time that my story, the way that I had to navigate pregnancy as a black, gay, trans man, is so different. Because I am black, there are a lot of systemic things I must deal with, then add being gay, then add being trans on top of that. It's not just a matter of learning, it is about actively taking in a diverse approach to your education and your work.

You can see it in the way that people show up. People flock towards white trans men. I really don't know what it is, maybe they are less scary than the big black men.

I became Instagram famous because I was attacked by a political figure and a lot of the people who follow me now came over to protect me. 'Poor black trans man needs protecting.' They won't feel the need to do as much for the white trans guys maybe. I really want to make sure that that is pointed out.

Allyship is also paying. I can't tell you how many times I have been approached and been asked to do things for free. The last time I tried to pay my rent cheque using exposure alone, it didn't go well, let me tell you. Especially when you are coming to me from a platform I know you are getting paid by. I had someone ask me to be in their documentary and they gave me a $20 gift card. They were so apologetic that it wasn't much, but I was just pleased they gave me something. If that is all you have, I get it. People often say they don't have the means and they still want me to work for free – major networks and huge companies for pregnancy and birth and so on. They take time, effort and education away from us and give nothing back. It's a slap in the face because you are taking my lived experience and telling me it's worth nothing. A lot of people come into my inbox saying, 'I just want to ask a quick question about...', and when I send them back the link to book a time through my website, with a list of my fees, they really turn their noses up at that. They want me to take time out, away from my family, my kids, me doing whatever it is that I am doing in my life, to educate them about my life, for free. They obviously think I am clever or important enough to ask me in the first place, but they won't pay me for that work. You cannot call yourself an ally if all you are doing is going around looking for free shit. You are bleeding an already oppressed group of people.

Sometimes even if people do pay – say they pay to come on one of my courses or something – and then they don't show up, they slide into my inbox asking for the recording. When I tell them that they must pay again, I get a huge kick back. I do 'pay what you can tickets' too, so some people have paid $5 to be there, some have paid $100. So, if it wasn't worth your time to make sure you were available or at your computer or even in the right time zone, then why do I have to hand over more of my property to you? If you go to Beyoncé, and you miss her concert, you can't hit her up like 'Hey B! You gonna give me the recording?' It doesn't work like that.

I also think that it is important for trans people to understand that other trans people don't owe them free jewels. I have had people message me just saying, 'How do I get pregnant?', and I don't know them from a can of paint! I'm like, 'Hi, how are you, my family is good, thanks for asking. What is your name!' Wow, it can be exhausting, especially the white trans people taking the work from black trans people and using it to make themselves money. I have seen white trans men taking ideas or literal words from our work and using that to do their work. It is reminiscent of what we see throughout history and throughout the world. Even someone like Elvis made a lot of his money and hits off the back of black work and music. I am not saying that their experience and words are not valuable. However, white birth workers need to understand the power that they have just from being white. White trans men need to understand that being trans alone doesn't mean that your plight is the same as my plight. Especially if they are passing. We do not have the same plight. There needs to be an allyship built from white trans people and black trans people. Just putting 'Black Trans Lives Matters' on Instagram is not enough. As a black person, I can't just be angry and black, I will lose followers. So, I have to find gentle ways to call this out. I can't just say, 'Hey, this isn't your lane.' That is something that really needs to be talked about more. I hate to make it so race based, but that is the way the world works.

To be an ally, it's about education on so many levels. It's education not just on white birthing people. Pushing for equality for black birthing bodies in the birthing world. Pushing for us to receive the same medical care. Without going down into trauma porn, let's push for black bodies to stop being offered abortions. I speak to white people and they aren't offered this.

There is no database for trans people of who is safe, who we can go to. I tell people all the time, it's okay to say that you are LGBT+ friendly. To me, it's very reminiscent of 'black-owned business' or, back in segregation, 'blacks welcome'. It sounds extreme but really that is what it feels like. Hopefully at some point we won't need this, but for now we really need to know who is safe and who will welcome us. Knowing that someone is putting in the work relieves so much anxiety for me straight off the bat, rather than thinking I must go in and do so much education with them straightaway. There is a fine line between showing their safety and doing it to advance their business and being tokenistic. When I think about having another kid, my first thoughts are, I don't live in New York City anymore. I live in Texas now. Where the hell would I go for care? That's the biggest anxiety for me. To have someone to say 'I took these courses' or 'I am doing the work' would help. Otherwise, how would I know who to go to?

Social media is life right now (in this pandemic). Make sure that you are following a plethora of people, not just white trans masculine people, so that you have a better, more well-rounded education. The trans community varies so much, you cannot just follow or know one trans person, read one book or listen to one podcast and know how to care for us. Not every trans person is qualified to educate you but at least try to expand who you follow.

If you work for an organization, like a doula school or midwifery school, push for them to do company-wide training so that you are all starting off on the right foot. There should be courses offered by trans people, about the trans experience of getting pregnant, pregnancy and birth.

*

Kayden continues this essential work in LGBT+ competency and visibility for black trans masculine people. He really is a gift to us all.

The Fox family: an interview with Caprice

I really wanted to go to Bristol to meet this amazing family in person, but as it often does, being a doula got in the way of travel plans, and being on call I couldn't cross the country to meet them. So, Caprice and I settled on a Zoom call.

I wanted to speak to Caprice because not only is she othered as a lesbian parent, but she is also othered as a black woman, and as a parent to a dual heritage child.

We spoke for nearly an hour and below is the conversation we had. I have omitted my words as Caprice's words are powerful enough alone.

For me personally, from such a young age, I knew that my purpose was to be a mother, to start a family. I've had other ambitions in life and in work of course, but I knew in my heart that this is what I was made to do.

I did resent in a way having an aspect of that taken away from me. We were quite hasty in getting rid of the donor information. We are my child's family, and we are her parents. She doesn't need this information, so I thought at the time. Since then, in speaking to other families and doing further soul searching, I have realized that it was hasty. She may have questions that she wants to peruse when she is older. That's her choice and right. I have the relevant numbers and codes that she needs, if she wants them, when she is older.

We tried artificial insemination first, at home with a donor we found online. However, because it was an at-home insemination it counted as a 'known' donor – not in the sense that we knew the person, but it wasn't anonymous.

The system isn't clear or accessible to everyone. People are writing their own contracts. That is something that we considered but we asked ourselves if we could protect ourselves and our child properly without getting legal advice and assistance. That is something that hetero parents don't even have to consider, that someone else might have a right to their child.

We had some awful questions from people. They were coming from a place of good, a place of love, but I found it so disrespectful. 'Did you get married just for the birth certificate?' NO! We got married because we are in love and wanted to cement our relationship, in a legal sense, in front of our friends and family.

What I would want to see changed is for medical professionals to be more educated. I think that it is such a huge issue that same-sex parents come across. So many people must educate their healthcare professionals, their midwives and so on with things that could make a really big difference to your experience, things that are so simple!

For example, how you would like to be referred to. Learning and knowing that these are the parents, not the biological mother and her partner. Learning the terminology. There is no dad, there is a donor. Or there is no mum, there is a surrogate. Those titles do not equate to parenthood. We came across this a few times and it's such a hard pill to swallow when you are both in such a vulnerable state of mind. You are already quite fragile. It needs to change.

We hadn't realized that when parents aren't married that the other parent didn't have any (legal) status, in the sense that they wouldn't be on the birth certificate. We were completely unaware of that. We did get married, but that wasn't the reason we got married, of course. However, then when we wanted to move forward with the process of starting a family, we were so relieved to know that we didn't need to worry about that side of things. After being in such a vulnerable state after giving birth, we didn't have to go to the council office and adopt our own child. That wasn't something that we had to worry about.

My wife suffered with postnatal depression. We are now able to call it that. She wasn't the biological parent, she didn't carry our daughter, but she did suffer.

There aren't many instances when we need to explain who the gestational parent is and who the non-biological parent is, but sometimes healthcare professionals need to know, so we use 'non-bio parent'.

We took part in a campaign with the NSPCC recently and they are doing a big push about perinatal mental health in both parents. Throughout our journey, because I had quite a difficult pregnancy, the professionals were very focused on me and my feelings. Sometimes during the appointments my wife didn't even have a chance to speak, let alone talk about her feelings, or discuss them at all. It was difficult. For the fourth trimester, she really struggled. It goes such a long way when people are aware of the feelings of both parents. It can make a huge difference in families' lives. If health visitors or the GP had been a little bit more encouraging or supportive, I don't know if she would have suffered; she may have, but maybe not to the same extent.

She was completely overlooked, until we had a new health visitor. It was so simple. She spoke to me and did everything she needed to do. Then she turned around and asked Holly, 'And how are you?' So simple! That opened the flood gates for her, so to speak. She was almost given permission to open and not feel ashamed or embarrassed that she was feeling this way. You are expected when the baby comes along to be overwhelmed with love and she felt so guilty about how she felt. She had no avenue or opportunity to let that out.

Thinking back to our initial consultation with our GP, she honestly just looked baffled the whole time. She did say, 'I don't have a lot of information; I will go away and do some research.' That's fine. She asked us to fill in a form. Immediately it said Mother/Father. We crossed that out. So, before we had even got into the service, before we'd got to the crux of the form, we were erased. We scoffed about it at the time but really that is something that has stuck with us. We went private in the end. It was so frustrating as we were told we had to show evidence that we were trying for a child 12 times before the NHS could offer us help. They did say, with a quiet undertone, 'If you want to, you could say you have been trying with your boyfriend for two and a half years.' I just glazed over at that point, as that was so insulting to us. There one hundred per cent should be a separate referral path for same-sex families. The checklist that the NHS has doesn't work for all families.

If you are in a hetero relationship and have polycystic ovary syndrome, low egg count, and so on, I know that you can get support on the NHS. As a lesbian woman (or bisexual person in a same-sex relationship) you cannot get that help. So, if you have two women with the same condition, one straight and one lesbian (or bisexual), they aren't offered the same treatment, the same options. That is the absolute definition of discrimination.

When we got to a clinic, the difference in the language was amazing. They were used to working with families who weren't cis, who weren't hetero. They were just educated and aware. I remember seeing another couple in the waiting room and the staff had made assumptions. The family must have said something, and I heard them saying, 'Oh sorry, how would you like to be referred to?' That was it. Done. So simple. Going forward they made no mistakes. It just makes such a big difference. It made us feel – and I hate to say the word – normal. They were excited, saying, 'Oh, you are both going to be mummies', just like they might call a man daddy and so on.

I have had people asking, 'Where is her dad?' And when I say she hasn't got a dad, they say 'Oh, is he one of them?' because we're black. They assume he is the stereotype of the not-present black dad. I've had that twice and I just couldn't believe it.

Also, I have had problems with people, from when she was quite young, wanting to touch her hair. You can't walk up to people and grab a part of their body. I really want to teach our daughter that her hair counts.

People need to learn about the history of what black people have been referred to: half caste, mixed and so on. Educate themselves a little bit. People aren't half caste; they aren't half of anything. That is a real bugbear. I experience it from all around. People say, 'It's so beautiful and wonderful to have half caste babies', 'They are so cute' and so on. This relentless objectification of dual heritage people makes me so uncomfortable. 'Do you think she will be one of "those" babies with dark skin and green eyes?' There is a whole movement on social media, like Facebook pages and Instagram, just objectifying babies. It's so strange. It is so, so wrong.

The other issue I come across daily is that black women are aggressive. It happens so much on social media. In my younger years, I would laugh it off and even friends would be like 'Oh, here comes the sassy black woman', clicking their fingers and waggling their heads about. I would laugh. As I've got older, and especially since becoming a mother, I know how damaging this is. I want our daughter to be able to grow up and voice her opinion. Be passionate, be angry, be loud if she wants to or needs to be.

*

I was taken aback by the Fox family's story. The simplest things did and could have made such a huge difference.

Simply being aware that you or your service might be caring for an LGBT+ person or couple can have such far-reaching benefits.

The people working in the fertility clinic didn't require expensive training or new computer systems or forms. They simply treated the Fox family as any other parents, and by slightly adjusting their language they made them feel safe, valued and protected.

Caprice's experience as a woman of colour and the mother to a dual heritage child is far from individual.

As well as working on our language and assumptions regarding LGBT+ people, we need to work on our language and assumptions of black and brown parents.

Mars Lord of Abuela Doulas writes in her blog[1] that part of the disparity that the MBRRACE report highlighted in 2017 showed us is that the assumptions people make about black women is this strong black woman stereotype. It means that black women are left in pain, are ignored, diminished and overlooked by healthcare professionals. If this is subconscious or not, it doesn't change the impact that it is having on the mortality rates in the UK. It's not pie. There is enough inclusion to go around.

Freddy McConnell: *Seahorse*

It was a very bright but chilly Wednesday in November when I got in my car to go to Kent to meet Freddy. You may or may not know Freddy from the documentary *Seahorse*,[2] shown on the BBC. Freddy is a journalist, trans rights activist and super cool dad.

Seahorse follows Freddy on his journey to fatherhood, from the early days of stopping T and waiting for his period to return, to his journey through using sperm donors in a London clinic. It ends with his beautiful birth, in the water. It's an event of pure power.

It brought many feelings for me. Mainly elation and joy at seeing, on my TV, at home, on the bloody BBC, a trans man give birth. Here he is in all his glory, birthing his baby like a fucking badass.

Love it.

Of course, there were parts that were hard to watch. Freddy's first

1   https://marslord.co.uk/doula/what-does-it-mean-to-silence-a-voice
2   https://seahorsefilm.com

attempt with a donor not being successful. The break-up of Freddy's relationship. The most poignant scene, in terms of my work and this book, was when Freddy went through the documents given to all women and birthing people by the NHS. The big book of 'notes' that you are told to carry with you always – it's massive, thanks for that!

We watch Freddy go through correcting the language to fit his experience. Removing words like maternity and replacing with paternity and so on. This struck me as an avoidable, quick, easy fix.

Also, there is the scene where Freddy is having dinner with his mum and her friends, family friends. This struck me as a beautiful intention of inclusivity. Towards the end of the sequence, we see Freddy almost zoning out with all the mention of 'women', 'woman', 'mums'. The topic turns to clothes and maternity clothes. Whether its editing or such, Freddy is talked over repeatedly about his choice of clothes, where to buy them, and that they aren't that 'feminine'. It's another heart-breaking but accurate example of how the needs and wants of the trans community can't be explained or reasoned by cis people. An example that cis women often feel as they can justify it by saying, 'I would wear them if they were men's or women's jeans', but that is a safety, a privilege that cis people have.

In another scene, we see Freddy walking along the sea front in his picturesque seaside town in Kent as he muses, 'If all men got pregnant then it would be taken so much more seriously.'

When I contacted Freddy on Instagram, I maybe naively thought that he wouldn't want to be in my book. He'd been in a film, and he was a journalist, a real person! He replied within a few minutes and told me how excited he was to be involved in the process and we set a date for a few weeks' time to meet in Kent and have a chat.

The following is a transcript of our discussion. I have omitted any non-relevant parts. Us talking about what cake to buy with our coffee probably wasn't interesting (I had a biscotti; he had a chocolate brownie).

I went with a few questions written down, but I really wanted Freddy to start talking and for me to listen. I didn't want to try and pre-empt too much. However, I also wanted to avoid asking the obvious. I am no journalist, and here I am trying to interview one. I am just a doula with a big gob and a passion for queer birth inclusion.

AJ: So, in the process so far, I haven't got a full set of questions that I've asked everyone, as that wouldn't work. Most of the focus of the book is about building awareness, but also, of course, to effect change. So, one of the main questions I've asked people in the process is: If you could say something to all healthcare professionals – so midwives, doctors, professionals that are in the birth and baby world – what, from your experience, would you want them to know?

Freddy: I would hope that on the most basic level I would feel reassured that everyone in that world knows that they could encounter someone like me. A trans person or a non-binary person. By having that level of awareness, it might never happen, there aren't many of us, but you are cutting out so much risk by just knowing it happens. Having that interpersonal experience where someone misgenders you is hard and that shouldn't happen. Hopefully one day that will never happen again to anyone. Having your life in these people's hands, and the life of your child, and when they aren't prepared on any level, that's unforgivable. I often think that people think this is just a matter of language and being respectful. We aren't just talking about that!

AJ: It's just that, it can be life and death. You spoke on the BBC previously about the dad in America who went to the emergency department and had pains and he told them 'I am pregnant' and their unpreparedness (for a trans man being pregnant) meant that help was delayed and the baby died!

Freddy: It must have been so traumatizing for the healthcare professionals as well, not to cheapen what he and his family went through. There are just so many levels of trauma that we need to and could quite easily cut out. With just that small level of awareness.

And I guess another thing is I want people to feel reassured that there is no extra magic or complicated set of skills that you need to know. If you are a midwife or person in that field, then you probably are going to be, or consider yourself, quite a compassionate person. Respectful and caring. All you need to do to be caring for trans and non-binary persons is just extend that a little.

It's nothing complicated or vastly different to what you are doing. It might feel unfamiliar, but work a little bit harder and you will so quickly get it and then you can just get on with your job of caring for people and everyone will just be happy and safe, and having a positive experience.

AJ: I think that's exactly right, it's not this huge upheaval. I think that the very minimum that people can do is memorize pronouns. But then, of course, ideally people need to go further and unpick their biases of the binary and trans rights and so on. I'm not saying that should be the goal, but that is the *bare* minimum that people can do.

Freddy: I imagine that when people are trained to be midwives, they are trained to respect the individual. Rather than treating them all the same, and not making assumptions about people. That's all that we (trans and non-binary people) are saying. Go away and do some learning but don't project that onto the person you are caring for now. Hopefully they will enjoy that process, of learning, but those are two different things.

AJ: It is an interesting point that you raise. So, in the doula world there is always talk that 'all options are valid' so that everyone gets to pick where they give birth, how they give birth, to decline induction or opt for water birth. We unquestionably – well, I hope, most doulas would unquestionably – support what their client chooses, but suddenly when that client is a trans or non-binary, we don't know what we are talking about. Why can we support some clients and not others?

Freddy: Exactly, most of your training should just carry over. So, don't feel worried, because if you feel worried, I'll feel worried. I am quite a people pleaser, so maybe my approach isn't assertive enough to be heard or something. But the main message I wanted to convey, to the midwife, was that I just wanted them to be at ease. Then I could be at ease. I didn't want to feel like there was any awkwardness, so I just really wanted to let them know that. Also, if they made mistakes, it was okay.

AJ: Yes! I think people are so scared of making mistakes that they don't try! I did a podcast yesterday for the plus-size pregnancy people. They asked what's the first thing we should know about pronouns and so on. And I said, 'That you are going to fuck it up.'

Freddy: One hundred per cent.

AJ: So, let's just deal with that now, let's get rid of the elephant in the room. You are going to misgender me, you are going to misgender other people. But if you are trying, then that's the important part. If you say you are trying but you consistently get it wrong with no improvement, then are you genuinely trying? I know it's decades of entrenched idiolect, so binary and heteronormative is going to tick over still for you. There is a huge difference between a violent misgendering and an accidental misgendering.

Freddy: Oh yes, one hundred per cent. When I think about people going home to practise, that's not for my benefit; if you want to get it right, and, someone suggests practising when you aren't in the company of the person, then that's for *your* benefit. If you then roll your eyes or say 'Oh, I don't want to do that' then *that* shows your intent. The best thing that people can do if they misgender me is to immediately apologize, and then let's move on. I find it so awkward.

AJ: It distracts from the importance of why it was wrong. 'Oh, I'm so sorry, I tried really hard' and now I feel bad that you feel bad. So, you have taken the issue, and made it about yourself, rather than about me. I don't think people are doing that because they are trying to manipulate the situation but now the focus is on them being hurt or sorry rather than trying to do better.

Freddy: And the media narrative on all this is that it is like punishable by death to misgender someone!

AJ: Yes, or you'll get banned from Twitter!

Freddy: No trans person has ever said I want it punishable by death. It's so unfair. Also, something that is particularly relevant to the world of being a doula is that is it correct to say that part of your scope is to make the person you are with feel at ease? They shouldn't feel uncomfortable.

AJ: Yeah of course, absolutely.

Freddy: So a part of that is not making it a big deal when you misgender someone, because then the client/doula relationship is flipped on its head because it shouldn't be the client who is being the doula because they have misgendered them.

AJ: As a healthcare professional or a doula, you can pay for this knowledge. There are courses run by Gendered Intelligence, you can buy this book, you can buy other LGBT books, you can watch films, you can watch *Seahorse*, you can watch *A Deal with the Universe*,[3] you can listen to podcasts by queer people. There are places to get this information from. You certainly shouldn't be asking for it from clients or patients.

Freddy: In a way, if someone fucks up and then corrects themselves and moves on, I will say that that deepens trust. Obviously, if someone never gets it wrong that's ideal. But it's like a mutual respect thing. You do the right thing. It demonstrates that you can acknowledge

---

3   A documentary that focuses on a trans masculine family and their journey to conception and parenthood.

mistakes you have made. That is rare in any context. Aside from misgendering, if someone can show to me that they had an opportunity to demonstrate this ability and take responsibility for their actions, deal with something like this well, I feel like I understand them as a person better.

AJ: I completely agree. It's comparable to when you have a consultation about the risks of something. Rather being told that the risk increases, without knowing the facts and figures, the studies behind it, I would prefer them to say 'hang on a minute', then get the correct information and tell me. That shows that they have your best interests at heart. That, in my opinion, builds trust.

Freddy: Yeah absolutely, all these things that show that someone is open and fair.

AJ: Absolutely. I agree! Shocker!

Freddy: [laughing] Yes, we are so unreasonable.

AJ: Tying into the point you made about the punishable by death argument. Some people say, 'Oh, you can't even ask for women-centred care anymore', 'We can't call it a women's hospital anymore', 'We can't use any gendered language at all!' That ties into, well, I can't say my favourite scene, because it was hard to watch, in *Seahorse* where you were going through the notes, crossing through the gendered language. I immediately felt that, as it's so important to what I do.

Freddy: Uh huh.

AJ: I am of the opinion that completely removing woman, women, feminine language and so on isn't the right thing to do. What is your opinion on removing feminine language?

Freddy: I'm glad you said that because I don't think that either.

Have you spoken to Helen Green in Brighton? They are a non-binary midwife.

AJ: Oh yes, actually I do think I know who they are. I think we are friends on Facebook (sorry Helen!).

Freddy: Well, they were at Trans Pride Brighton and that was where I first met them. They were telling me about the forms that they were creating, to have an alternative to the standard pregnancy forms. So, Helen and their team, their way of working is that they are additive, which means that none of what they are doing is meant to replace what already exists. I'm not sure exactly how that would work in practice. I'm not saying that *everyone* must have difference forms because of me, but that there is an alternative, so that I and other people who are pregnant can get a set of forms that are appropriate to us. I mean, it might sound like we are creating an endless variety of forms, but I don't think that is the case. Because ninety-nine per cent of the time you can use the form that already exists. You just need a very small box of gender-neutral language forms.

AJ: Some trans men may need reassurance and affirmations of masculine language.

Freddy: Yeah absolutely. I just wonder, in the long term, I can't think of many downsides of having everything as gender neutral. Right know, I don't want to bring the 'heat' on to non-binary people that that would create.

AJ: So, if there was no 'heat' would that be your suggestion?

Freddy: Yeah. That goes across society in general. I think that in all healthcare contexts, you can use anatomically correct language like breast tissue. If someone can show me an example of where it would be dangerous to use gender neutral language, then I will be open to hearing that and having my mind changed. My general feeling is that in maybe 50 or 100 years' time, all the official documentation could just be gender neutral.

So, in my court case (to be recorded as the father of my baby), we are asking for parent or father. Because I am a parent, I have no argument with that. I think that the gendering of parenting is damaging. The sense of sexism, it's damaging and limiting to women, it restricts men from nurturing and caring potential. As a father, I am fully capable of doing all those things.

I would just love for there to be some forms that I can use that don't make me feel erased, where I don't have to go through and correct them. It's mentally very taxing. When I was pregnant, a friend of mine who was pregnant at the same time, another trans man, described it as like a 'chip, chip, chip' away every day of your resilience.

AJ: Like microaggressions. Like a dripping tap?

Freddy: Can you count it as a microaggression if it's just on a form?

AJ: I would say you can because it's that constant poke or prod at your existence; something that could pass a lot of people by without them noticing. So, in the general ether of the world, people wouldn't notice. Like a feminist might notice where the patriarchy is holding women back, in those 'micro' instances, but say a cis man might not. I would say a microaggression is something that takes a tiny piece off each time. So maybe on its own, if that was the one thing to happen to you, you might be able to shrug it off and carry on. When it is this constant barrage of microaggressions, it adds up to a huge problem.

Freddy: Yes definitely. I think that I worry slightly. I don't want it to seem a part of that chipping away that comes from everything about pregnancy being about women. Because I don't want to suggest that any of that is negative. It's not meant to be, it's all meant to be there. I'm not saying that it's okay that it carries on that way. It felt like there was a lot of stuff that I was having to encounter every day that was wearing me down. A lot of it would be microaggressions but a lot of it was also, like, undefinable. Just kind of in the ether, too hard to pin down. Yeah, it was just hard for me. Again, that becomes a safety thing. Say if you (a trans or non-binary person) were worried about something and you googled it, and everything was erasing you at every line, every word, then you might choose not to read it.

AJ: We already know through the NHS and Stonewall studies that trans people are less likely to seek medical attention due to the fear or experience of transphobia. So, if we ring the birthing unit and we hear 'women's clinic' or 'mother and baby unit', it is possible that that could be enough for someone to disengage with those services! We can't overlook a whole community just because it's a small percentage, when the costs are so high. One of the examples in my book is a lesbian couple who, every time they went to see a healthcare professional, were asked, 'Is this your sister, your friend, your mother?' That's a healthcare professional telling them that it's much more likely in my mind that you are sisters, friends or mother, daughter and grandchild than it is likely that you are a family.

Freddy: Oh god.

AJ: So that again comes back to the point that healthcare professionals need to be aware that we exist. It is possible that you will care for us and a big burly guy with a beard is going to come in, in labour.

Freddy: Big and burly pregnant men! It's a beautiful thing!

AJ: But we've had trans men refused access to maternity units until 'mum' arrives. So, they are in labour in a hospital corridor, trying, between contractions, to 'explain themselves' and justify their presence.

Freddy: Who is that keeping safe? That's the whole thing! We're not asking to reinvent the wheel. It's just making the space slightly bigger.

AJ: That's always my argument, that I've never said that women don't give birth. Ninety-nine per cent of the time that's going to be correct. How does it hurt to say on a form, for example, 'The woman OR pregnant person'? No one can ever answer that.

Freddy: Absolutely. When people say 'Oh you can't say that' or 'You can't say this' I just have to question the intent behind that statement. Who is saying that you can't say that? Why would you? If you need to have that language, if you need to exclude people, who you are being told exist, who we know exist, then should we have to demonstrate our humanity, our existence? What do we have to do to prove to you that we deserve inclusion? You are using that as a cover for some opinion or feeling that you have.

AJ: It's reminiscent of the tabloids saying, 'You can't even fly the Union Jack anymore!'

Freddy: Yeah, it's political correctness gone mad! What are the real issues here? What are you worried about? If you are worried, then let's talk about it. It's important to talk about it. If you have concerns, they can almost certainly be allayed. Unless it's bigotry. Unless it's prejudice. Then, sorry, we can't help you.

AJ: That makes so much sense because people are always saying, 'We can't even talk about this.' I say: No! If you are acting like a bigot, and a homophobe or a transphobe, you are going to get shot down. If you ask a genuine question, and you ask it in an appropriate setting, and in a way that is not violent or bigoted, then we can have a conversation. Again, the pressure to be 'nice' is put onto the oppressed people – the queer.

Freddy: The whole argument that you must be nice just doesn't add up. There is no cost or, like, social penalty for excluding trans people. So the whole idea that you can't say this or that is just wrong. No one has ever had any cost levied against them for being mean or discriminatory. If someone in a minority community speaks up and demands equality, then they often are excluded or rejected. Even worse but in a vulnerable situation. So again, I've got no time for it.

AJ: Going back slightly to the microaggressions, there was a part in *Seahorse* where we see an example of cis straight people thinking they understand what we are asking for, when they haven't got a clue. There is a scene where you are having dinner with your mum and family friends and they are talking about jeans and they say, 'I would wear them if they were men's or women's jeans.' The person seems so sweet and loving, but that is a great example to me that cis straight people can't relate to, or compare, expectations of gender roles or expression.

Freddy: That is a powerful scene. I had no idea when it was being filmed what it was really capturing. The experience I was having was one of real discomfort, just wanting to hide away. I had no sense that it was coming across on the camera.

AJ: The way it pans out, you are just nervously laughing and still. It made my heart ache.

Freddy: It was like, all I can do is just sit here. Yeah, it is a good demonstration of how someone can be saying something, but not realize what they are saying. There was no malice whatsoever. I think in that sense it was important to have in there. I don't think it could ever give the impression that it is okay. It's a good antidote to the idea that everyone must get everything right, or there would be this massive showdown.

AJ: I really don't want it to seem like an attack on the person who said those things. You can hear and see how much love is in the room – the love they all have for you. However, it's an example that your intent doesn't negate your impact. I think it's a good thing for people who want to be allies to see that.

Freddy: Absolutely, that's why I wanted it in there. That's why I wanted to make the film at all. For people to experience something that they, statistically speaking, won't. Again, there aren't a lot of trans people. There are even fewer who are pregnant. That might change as we go forward.

AJ: Oh, it's going to change. One of the statistics in the book shows that there is a 15–20 per cent rise, year on year, of lesbians registering babies. More people are coming out as queer, gender queer, gender non-conforming and trans. So, yeah, it's absolutely going to change.

Freddy: We really need doctors to stop telling us trans men that taking testosterone will make us infertile. There is so much anecdotal evidence that that isn't true. There was no evidence in the first place to even say it. It was about some weird insurance policy.

That scene (about the jeans) was so powerful. It was such an unusual thing to have shown. With all the visibility that trans and non-binary people...I was going to say enjoy but...

AJ: [laughing] Yeah, not all of it we enjoy.

Freddy: Oh my god [laughing]. It's mainly a liability. It brings so much heat on us, which we don't want. Despite there being so much of it, it is rare just to have any level of nuance explained. That scene has so much nuance in it. There is so much going on. So much love in that room. I was so naive about how I would feel in that room. Now looking back, like mate, did you even think? Did either of us think? I should have known by that point that it generally made me uncomfortable when cis women tried to relate to my experience. I guess I didn't even think I would end up being asked that question: will you be going by mum or dad?

AJ: It struck me that it wasn't an open question. I always give the example that we ask that question all the time: preferred names or pronouns. When I worked as a sling librarian, someone would come with their parent(s) and it was so easy to say, 'Hi grandma, or do you go by nanny or nan?', and so on. There was no awkwardness. You would just say, 'Oh, right, granny it is.' We move on! We already do it in that sphere, in that context. Why is it so hard to transfer it to parents?

Freddy: Exactly. After that evening, you don't see it in the film. We met up for coffee and, although painful at the time, it opened the conversation and brought us much closer. My mum's friend is now firmly my friend. We are so close. They are close to my son. We really used that as a learning opportunity. In the long run, when the camera wasn't there anymore, she totally understood why it was uncomfortable for me. I think she really, really struggles with the fact that it is in the film to some extent. It's better for her now. I am so thankful that she was able to sit with that discomfort, to let it be. Ultimately, she realized how powerful that scene was.

AJ: I was a little bit worried about bringing that up. It's such a loving scene, so full of love. I didn't want it to feel like I was attacking her.

Freddy: No, no, not at all. No one has ever said or done that. She came when my son had to have his tongue tie snipped, which happened late because I wasn't chest-feeding and so we got not so great care, even though I knew, as his parent, that he needed it done. That friend of ours came with us and was there for us.

AJ: That's wonderful. Tongue tie is another soap box I could climb up on for a good few hours.

Freddy: Me too!

AJ: [laughing] Let's not do that.

Freddy: [laughing] No, no, let's not do that. That's the power of the film, though.

AJ: It's subtle but it's clear. It's well done.

Freddy: Yes, thank you. That scene is also a great example of how *anyone* can do that. She's not in the queer world. She's just my mum's friend. It just proves that it doesn't take any special knowledge. All it takes is caring about someone, having that empathy. Hopefully the film gives people the opportunity to feel. If you aren't trans, you are never going to know what that feels like. However, if someone you love is trans, then as my friend showed, if you go at it with love, anyone can get there and be supportive and loving.

AJ: That's the important part. We know that the statistics and risks of suicide go down when trans and non-binary people are supported. When people use their chosen name and pronouns and so on, it's not just polite or placating, it is life saving.

Freddy: Oh absolutely, and it's so easy to do.

Steph: intersex and pregnant

Steph reached out to me on Instagram after I shared a post during LGBT+ History Month in 2021 about what intersex means. She was so happy to see inclusion for intersex people she kindly agreed to talk to me about her experiences as an intersex wheelchair user who is in the early stages of pregnancy with her partner, Alex.

I spoke to Steph over Zoom in February 2021.

Steph: I am a travel blogger, that is what I do, but I am intersex, I have hormonal changes. I use she/her pronouns and I have a condition where I produce way too much testosterone.

I have had an interesting background with medical professionals all my life. As most intersex people will tell you, most of our experiences aren't that great. We're often subjected to horrific experiences as children. Our opinions and voices aren't really considered. A lot of the time, healthcare professionals will say to the parents that we need to do XYZ (operations or hormone treatments) because the child doesn't completely fall into the binary options of sex. Things like surgery and hormones at such a young age can cause so many problems down the line. Things like urinary tract infections (UTIs) are quite common. I have reoccurring UTIs still today, because of the surgeries I had to go through when I was really young. I also have a lot of difficulties with hormones as I was put on them at nine years old.

AJ: Hormone replacement therapy?

Steph: Yeah. I was put on oestrogen and progesterone when I was nine.

AJ: Woah, nine!

Steph: Yeah, people just don't even realize that this happens, and they hardly consider the wishes of the children either. They tell you, this medicine will make you better. It got so bad that at 14 my gran got parental responsibility for me and took me to the GP to try and get me off all these medications. She said that if at 18 you want to go back on them then that's fine, but I didn't want to be on them. The GP was amazing and said, 'I can't tell you to stop but if Steph wants to stop then I can't stop her.' I am really concerned that now I am pregnant, that those hormones could be affecting me.

It's a strange time, because I am trying to learn to trust healthcare professionals with me and my baby, when I have grown up not being able to trust them. All that I have been through, the medical trauma of it all. It is very real in the intersex community, so many people go through it.

AJ: It must be so hard, because so many people when they are pregnant don't feel 'believed'. It's like this cultural thing maybe, but a lot of people I have supported haven't been believed that they are in labour, for example, so you have to trust the healthcare professionals, with all your past trauma of them not listening to you.

Steph: Yes! That is a fair summary of how many intersex people feel.

My midwife is amazing, I must say. She did pre-warn me that child-birth and being pregnant might trigger my PTSD from the treatment I experienced as a child. It was great that she warned me. This was at my eight-week booking appointment, so I knew I had seven months to prepare myself, educate myself and give myself the best chance of having a positive experience. I am looking into hypnobirthing as well.

AJ: That makes so much sense. It really drives home why all birth work-ers need to be LGBT+ competent. I teach quite a lot of hypnobirthing instructors and some people question why they need to be informed, or why others who aren't present at birth or aren't healthcare profes-sionals need to be LGBT+ competent. That's a poignant example of how if a hypnobirthing teacher or school isn't LGBT+ inclusive, those who could really benefit from their products and services could miss out by not being made to feel welcomed, valued, and safe with them.

Steph: Yes, that's the thing. I brought this up with my midwife. My other half noticed it first. I handed him all the leaflets that they gave me, and he started flicking through and immediately he said, 'Oh god, they need to change the language in these leaflets! It's really not inclusive at all!' So, I mentioned it to my midwife and she said it is something the trust is trying to get sorted. I mean I use she/her pronouns, so it doesn't affect me too much. My other half, bless his heart, just said it was another example of why he couldn't compre-hend carrying a child, after everything he had been through. Which is why I am doing it!

AJ: How have you found being intersex, a wheelchair user and part-ner to a trans man throughout the process of conception and early pregnancy?

Steph: Ah, the usual comments and questions. I did have a friend message me and do the classic 'Can I ask you a personal question? Is yours and Alex's kid a sperm donor baby?'

AJ: Mmm, that's a common one. I get that sometimes, particularly when healthcare professionals may have to ascertain how this baby was conceived, to rule out risk factors and the like.

Steph: Yep, I completely get that.

AJ: What I usually say is it's not that you can't ask those questions…

Steph: [finishing my sentence because we are firm friends at just 13 minutes into our conversation!] …it's *how* you ask it.

AJ: Exactly. Love it! I talk about language, assumptions and delivery. So, you need to have the language to ask the questions, rather than making assumptions, and you also need the bedside manner – not sure if that is the right expression – or the sensitivity to ask those questions in the right way. But only when it is essential to know to help give the best care for the pregnant person or the baby.

Steph: Yes, that all makes perfect sense.

AJ: So, what advice, or what do you want to give healthcare professionals about asking these, what are perceived as 'difficult', questions?

Steph: What I say to most people is that when you need to ask a question, think before you speak. Think about how you are going to ask it. Don't make assumptions. Once you make those assumptions it's like a barrier. When we are perceived as a cis couple, and it's clear the healthcare professional has made that assumption, it does make us think before answering freely. We aren't sure if they are a safe person we can tell everything about ourselves, you know?

AJ: I do, yes, I do.

Steph: My midwife was great at this. She said, 'Before we start, is there anything you want to tell me about you?' Straightaway, because she had asked this open question and left it to me to tell her what I knew was relevant, it made me feel so at ease. Had she just assumed I was cis, and Alex was cis, then it would have come up further down the line and it would have put the emphasis on her to ask more questions. This way was so much easier and felt safer to me because I was in control.

AJ: Yeah, that's the difference between open questions and closed questions. Asking what you want, or need to tell me about you, what information you think I need to give you the best care that I can. As opposed to telling me about your sexuality, gender and so on. Sometimes I call it 'the drop-down box paradox' because you are trying to ask the right questions to put everyone in these boxes and not everyone fits inside them.

Steph: Yeah! I said to the midwife on the phone when I called up, I said, my booking appointment needs to be longer, it's not going to happen in an hour. We need more time, with my medical history and my family's medical history.

AJ: The world would be so boring if we all fitted into the same boxes. I would hope that healthcare professionals reading this feel really empowered by this explanation. That it is not something overly complicated or that requires additional training. It is just giving the pregnant person space, time and opportunity to tell you what they need to tell you.

Steph: Yes, totally true.

AJ: Okay, well that's that bit sorted! That's one thing we've fixed! Would you mind telling me about your experience of accessing fertility treatment?

Steph: When we wanted to start fertility treatment, I knew I would need medication. With my medical history and exposure to hormones,

I knew that is what I would need to do to get my body in the right position. I went to my GP and said I needed a referral to the fertility team. They looked at me a bit confused and asked me to explain further. I said all you need to know is that my partner and I want to have a baby and we know that we will need assistance to make that happen.

The way we had decided that we would start trying is by me going on clomid (a medication used to treat infertility in women and those assigned female at birth who do not ovulate). We knew we would need this to get me into a cycle so I could ovulate. We were then going to do sperm donation privately. We had done a lot of research. Well, my partner had done a lot of the research. I just left most of that to him, and I focused on getting through all the assessments needed to get on the right medications and pathways to get assistance.

I did request not to be sent to my local hospital. That is the one that I have been under since I was a child and I have a lot of trauma associated with that building. I can't stand the medicalization of intersex people, and I knew I didn't want to go to my appointments there. I don't like to call (my intersex condition) a health condition, it's just a difference. People assume if you are intersex, you are a medical emergency. If you don't conform to what a 'normal' baby girl is or a 'normal' baby boy. Some people don't find out until puberty and they are very quickly put on hormones and surgeries are suggested. So, I knew I couldn't go to that hospital. Don't send me there. I can't do it.

AJ: Yep, I see that.

Steph: When I went to the clinic, I told them everything about me and what I thought I needed. They were trying to push me to go straight to IVF. I really wanted to try to do it at home with our donor. I knew we might have to (try IVF in the clinic) but I really wanted to try it at home so we could use our donor.

AJ: Did they not offer IUI first? Just straight to IVF?

Steph: Yeah, straight to IVF. They were worried that even with clomid I wouldn't ovulate. That was their biggest concern. I figured we might as well try it, see how far we got and then adjust our plan if it was needed. We were successful in May 2019. Unfortunately, we lost that baby. I was at Pride when I started miscarrying.

AJ: Oh, love...

Steph: It was awful because I was away from home and my partner was away working. I go to the local hospital with my notes and the first thing they read is that I am intersex. Straightaway they were saying things like 'You shouldn't have even been able to get pregnant in the first place!?' 'You won't ever be able to carry to term.'

AJ: As you went into A&E, experiencing a miscarriage, this is what they were saying to you?

Steph: Yep, as soon as they saw my notes and discovered I was intersex.

AJ: [stunned silence]

Steph: I did put a complaint in.

AJ: Fucking hell, Steph!

Steph: So, as I am having a miscarriage, they are telling me that this would have always happened and that I shouldn't try again, basically. I asked them what they think caused it, and they said it's because you are intersex.

AJ: [more stunned silence]

Steph: I screamed the hospital down to be honest. They didn't want me to leave because they were worried about me, obviously, but I just had to get off that ward. Immediately. I needed fresh air, I needed outside, I needed away from them.

AJ: Fucking hell, that's hideous.

Steph: So then once we had healed from that experience, we decided to try again... [laughing] During a pandemic!

AJ: Take the easy route, eh?

Steph: [laughing] We didn't even know if it was possible to do it during a pandemic, but the time felt right for us as a couple now that we had healed from our loss. I am now 11 weeks! I've had a scan, well, I have had more scans already than most people have during their whole pregnancy.

AJ: Oh gosh!

Steph: Yeah, I've had a lot of input from the early pregnancy unit. They were so sweet. So enthusiastic! All my blood tests are fine. I ended up crying with happiness at one of the scans because they said everything looks normal, your blood tests are fab, and it just felt so healing after being told it was my body that 'let us down' previously. Now here we are, and everything is going well.

AJ: Mate! That is amazing.

Steph: Yeah, they had made contingency plans for if my hormones dipped and they always framed it as: 'If you want to, you could try this', 'If we need to, we can offer you this.' It wasn't like at A&E at all. It was very open, and I really felt that they were offering me what they could, and it was me in control of what route we took.

AJ: Completely contrary to your previous experience as an intersex person with healthcare professionals then?

Steph: Pretty much, yeah. It was amazing. I felt in control of my hormone medications. As an intersex person that can be really empowering. It might also apply to trans or non-binary people as well. Give the person all the information they may need to know so they can access it and decide what is best for them.

AJ: Has that extended to your choices for pregnancy, birth and labour? I know it's a way off right now, but have you been given lots of choices and options? Or have you felt restricted because of your intersex condition or because you used home insemination?

Steph: Well, I am on a high-risk pathway, but not because of home insemination, because of my medical history. That is quite scary, but I do appreciate that because I get to have more scans, so I get to see my baby more.

AJ: That's the important thing is that you are happy with that, isn't it? I was high risk for both of my pregnancies because I had gestational diabetes.

Steph: Ah! I am high risk for that. I've got to have my glucose tolerance test soon.

AJ: Well, if you want to talk to someone who has been through it then you know where I am. I've got you!

Steph: Ah good to know, thank you!

AJ: I declined some of the extra scans with my second baby because it felt too intrusive as I was diet controlled, but then there are people, like yourself, who relish and appreciate that. It comes back down to choice and personal preference, doesn't it?

Steph: Especially with people who have previous medical trauma, for sure.

AJ: How have the people you have dealt with so far treated your partner?

Steph: Well, he hasn't been to any appointments in the hospital because of Covid. However, because that midwife asked me, at the outset, is there anything you want to tell me, I had told them from the start that Alex is trans. So, they have all been aware he is transgender and that is why we have used donor sperm. When we have had phone appointments he has been there on the phone with me, and they have needed to ask him any questions, they have done the same as they did with me. They asked open questions and allowed us to fill them in on what was relevant. They really allowed him that space to talk about his concerns and questions.

We did know from the outset, because of my medical history, that I would be on consultant-led care, so it didn't come as a shock for us.

AJ: The takeaway message I am hearing for healthcare professionals is that by your midwife asking these open questions and really giving you space to build up that trust, she has fostered this environment that you can trust her even given your past traumas and complexities.

Steph: Yeah, she has been there for every single appointment as well. With all the different scans and the consultant phone calls, she has been there with us.

AJ: Have you got a one-to-one midwife? Case loading?

Steph: Yep.

AJ: Oh, look at my shocked face that you feel safe and trust your healthcare professionals!

Steph: Yeah, I've got one-to-one!

AJ: Is that standard in your trust to have one-to-one midwives if you have certain...complexities – is it okay to say complexities?

Steph: Yeah, that's totally fine, it is complex! In our trust if you are high risk you go to one-to-one care.

AJ: That's amazing!

Steph: They have explained that in an emergency, obviously, I might have to switch, but I have met all the team leaders and other members of the one-to-one team, so I would feel safe with any of them.

AJ: That is fabulous! The things that you have explained that have enabled you to feel safe, cared for and listened to, these aren't huge differences.

Steph: It's just a switch of mindset. If you ask closed questions, you aren't going to be able to build that trust. If you ask open questions, they will feel more comfortable to tell you, and to divulge things to you over time. It's not something you need to do loads of training for, it's just a mindset.

Alex and I had this conversation the other day, about asking questions and talking about LGBT+ status and how, because of our age (22 and 27), we are like the last generation that went through school when Section 28 was a thing.[4]

AJ: Yeah!

Steph: So, all the midwives – well most of them – were in school when you couldn't ask questions freely.

AJ: Yeah, that is a good point!

---

4 Section 28, brought into law in 1988, made it illegal for local authorities to promote homosexuality.

Steph: Just because you didn't learn when you were younger doesn't mean you can't learn now.

AJ: That's a great sound bite! I might just call the whole book that!

Steph: [laughing] It's true though, isn't it? You can start doing your own independent learning and understanding. It's just understanding and mindset. Thinking before you speak. My midwife didn't make any assumptions about my disability either. Given that I was in a wheelchair at my appointments she didn't say 'This is what you will need' or 'This is what we normally do for folks in wheelchairs', she just asked me, 'With regards to your disability, do I need to know anything?'

AJ: Who is this midwife? I want her to be everyone's midwife, she sounds amazing.

Steph: She is incredible. She didn't just assume, for once, a healthcare professional didn't just assume, that I needed a hoist, which is a common misconception for wheelchair users. She also gave me the option of having appointments at home. She asked me if I would prefer that she didn't say I had to. Again, she gave me the choice.

AJ: That is fantastic. Thank you so much for sharing all of that with me, I really think it will be so helpful for people to read your experience and learn from that. Is there anything else we haven't covered that you think we should talk about, or that the people who care for pregnant people need to understand?

Steph: Everything we have talked about really. Just ask open questions rather than assuming you know the questions to ask. If you foster that open environment, it may be of benefit further down the line when you need to ask more questions. That person will feel more comfortable with you and may find it easier to talk to you about their concerns and can trust you.

I just want to thank you as well, AJ, for including intersex people in your LGBT+ History Month posts. I was like 'OH MY GOD, THANK YOU!' So many people forget us. We are almost like the forgotten sub-community. I don't know why.

AJ: The most common explanation I get for that is that people think it's so rare, and that it is an 'abnormality'. The first thing I learned when I started reading and listening to intersex people is that...

Steph: [finishing my sentence again because we are BFF now] It's not that rare!

AJ: It's not rare! And even if it was 'rare', it doesn't mean that intersex people are broken or an abnormality. It's only an abnormality if you assume that the whole world can be put, neatly, into two distinct boxes.

Steph: Exactly!

AJ: The other 'argument' I hear for not including intersex people in discussions around the LGBT+ community – particularly transgender people – is that you can't use intersex people to 'justify' trans people.

Steph: Oh my god! That is a whole thing, a whole can of worms! At Brighton Pride, of all places, I heard someone saying, 'Kids are too young for hormones', so I said, 'Would you say that about intersex kids?'

AJ: It's almost like you can only have hormones if 'we' are trying to 'fix' you.

Steph: Yep. Bang on. It is further complicated for people who are intersex and trans. They are told they can't have the hormones or surgeries that they need because of what they were subjected to as children. When I talk to people about letting intersex children make those decisions for themselves when they are older, people don't understand why I am so passionate about it. The interventions they are doing on intersex children aren't reversible in some cases.

AJ: Yeah, that is awful.

Steph: You can only give hormones to kids when you are trying to 'correct' them into the presumed gender binary.

AJ: Lots to think about here. Thank you again so much for your time and for sharing this with me. I know it's going to be so helpful to everyone reading this.

Steph: You're so welcome.

*

Steph and her partner's story really reminds us of the complexities of identities and intersectionality. I hope it will serve as a tangible example of why assumptions about the physical abilities of the bodies of those we care about can be so harmful, and how, with small, considered changes, we really can make the world of difference to families like Steph and Alex. Steph and Alex welcomed their beautiful baby in August 2021.

Laura-Rose Thorogood: sperm donation

I met Laura through Instagram when she messaged me from her incredible account for her organization, The LGBT+ Mummies Tribe. Considering I had a lowly under-1000 followers Instagram account, she was super sweet in sharing and sending people my way. The first time we talked it was like speaking to an old friend. As we both hailed from Essex, there was a geographic cultural understanding as well as an LGBT+ community understanding between us.

I knew I had to speak to Laura about her experience of being a lesbian who campaigns for access, support and funding for same-sex families, as well as her lived experience of having two children and being pregnant with her and her wife's third child.

AJ: Thank you so much for making the time to come talk to me, I know how busy you are, being pregnant and in the middle of a pandemic! I really appreciate you.

Laura: No worries at all, lovely; this is important and I am excited to be a part of it!

AJ: Bless you! So, this book, I hope, will be read by healthcare professionals as well as parents or intended parents who pick it up looking for more information and stories of solidarity. I have been asking people to tell me what they want the healthcare professionals to know. I see my role as guide, or narrator maybe, stringing together the stories of those with lived experience, using my own knowledge and expertise to join up the dots and make it impactful for the reader.

Laura: Yep, I get it, sounds great.

AJ: With that in mind, what do you want the healthcare professionals to know? What would you tell sonographers, midwives, doulas and so on about caring for someone who is having a baby via sperm donation?

Laura: Because we (The LGBT+ Mummies Tribe) do so much work with the NHS as well as my personal lived experience, I think this might be a long answer!

AJ: I don't mind that; you talk, and I'll listen.

Laura: Assumptions can be frustrating. Say sonographers, for example, you go in for a scan and rather than asking you who you are with today, they'll just assume that my wife is my mum, my friend, my sister before they consider it is possible that she is my wife.

AJ: Yep, almost every lesbian couple I have spoken to says this.

Laura: It's not just the sonographers of course, we've had it so many times over the last nine years. That could just be avoided by asking open questions. We've even had someone ask if this is my nana! In the end, my wife, understandably, got really annoyed. There are only four years between us. It is like it's not even conceivable that we could be a married couple. They just go straight for the relation assumption first.

AJ: Yeah, an open question would eliminate the risk of that straight-away, wouldn't it?

Laura: Yes. It happened throughout our first two pregnancies, and the one thing about being pregnant in a pandemic is that she can't come with me, so at least we aren't dealing with this at every appointment. I suppose that is the one good thing. She did come to one appointment this time round, and they didn't assume. I think the only reason that happened is because one of the healthcare professionals was gay. They just asked, 'Who have we here today?'

They also always assume I go by 'mum'. They shouldn't be assuming that I am a mum, I could be non-binary, I might be trans! I could go by something different. Many LGBT+ parents choose different names, so that is also frustrating. I could also be a surrogate and calling me mum could be really upsetting for me or for the intended parents. You just can't make these assumptions as they can be so harmful and detrimental to someone's mental health.

When they do this at the start of the appointment it puts us on the back foot. We feel like they haven't taken the time to understand us properly or our family dynamic, so they can best support us. It means we are trying to play catch-up with them almost, and it doesn't feel reassuring. The work we do with the NHS means we get it; we understand how much pressure the NHS is under and how little time they have for these appointments, but it doesn't take two seconds to ask an open question.

AJ: It's probably quicker than running through all the family members they can think of that might explain who this other person is with you. It's probably much quicker to ask, to be honest, isn't it?

Laura: Yes, that's true, it is quicker. Even if you think these people look like a heterosexual couple, you can't assume. You can't know that until you have asked the question.

AJ: Of course, yeah that assumption about who we are to each other is on top of another assumption of who we are biologically to the baby, as well as who we are emotionally to the baby. It's a whole thing.

Laura: So, when we explained to the sonographer who we were, we would say, I am the bio mum or she is the bio mum, or whatever the situation might be. We explained our experience which was that I am the gestational mum and we used in utero insemination (IUI) to get pregnant. Ninety-eight per cent of the people we encountered didn't know what IUI was. Not only that, but the role of being a non-biological mother is a difficult one. The lack of visibility and understanding, even down to how you are addressed, can have a real impact on people's journey to parenthood. When it should be a positive and exciting time. We had to spend so much time explaining to them, and they thought it was the same as IVF. I felt awkward for them because, surely, they should know what IUI is? It's not just LGBT+ people who require fertility treatment to have a family.

AJ: Wow, what? They didn't know what IUI is?

Laura: It was tiring for us to have to explain, and also we were wasting our time and their time and felt guilty for wasting NHS time and money. It wasn't just the sonographers though, most of the midwives we dealt with would say, 'Is that like IVF?' Before we got started in most appointments, we spent so long explaining, who we were, how we got pregnant, what IUI is, that it did become quite repetitive each time. At that time, we didn't have continuity of carer, so we always saw a different healthcare professional each time.

Then when we mentioned the donor, they would ask, 'Have you got medical history of the dad?', and we would have to say 'donor' multiple times until they started getting it. People are generally apologetic when they get it wrong. To be honest, I do feel sorry for the midwives and the other healthcare professionals who don't get the level of basic education that is required to support LGBT+ parents. It isn't their fault that they don't know this. Therefore, we do so much work with the NHS to try and impact change and improve the amount of education that people get around fertility treatment and LGBT+ paths to parenthood – not just for LGBT+ people but for cis and het people who don't have a straightforward path to pregnancy too.

AJ: I always say that it's not just LGBT+ people who will benefit, it's het people who use donors or surrogates too!

Laura: Right! It should be a mandatory part of training. Even if they do get some training, it's often a PowerPoint that hasn't been updated in years. We don't blame them because it isn't their fault that they haven't had this training. There are some who will continue to use 'dad' even after we have corrected them and explained. It does tend to be a particular demographic of midwives that continue to do it. You get the impression that this is because they will always consider the donor to be 'dad', because they are biologically the other half of the child. People make mistakes and it might slip out because that is what they are so used to saying and I can understand it to a certain extent in those circumstances. But it really hurts people, language is powerful. It takes energy and trust away from us every time they do it. Even thinking about het cis men, who are infertile, sitting there with their partners when they are pregnant using a donor or IVF and so on, and the midwife keeps referring to the donor as 'dad', how must that feel to them?

AJ: Yeah, it could be really destroying, couldn't it?

Laura: Yep, you could be really impacting someone's mental health for a couple or individual who have taken years and years, or thousands of pounds, and suffered loss, to get to this point. It is so crucial that language assumptions are addressed.

When we had our first child, the next day when the obstetrician was checking her over was a painful experience. She asked for Mum, so I went in with her and the baby. Then she called me Stacey, which is my wife's name, so I corrected her and said, 'I am Laura. I am her other mum.' I saw it on her face when she realized who I was, when she realized that I was gay. I just saw this look of disgust wash over her and she waved at me dismissively, telling the nurse assisting to take me away saying, 'I want the mum; I want the real mum. Get me the real mum.'

AJ: Woah!

Laura: At the time, this was nearly seven years ago when it happened, there wasn't a community like ours, and yours, where other LGBT+ parents might have warned us that this might happen. Or where you could listen to other people's lived experiences as a non-bio mother or parent. If it does happen though, there are some ways of dealing with it. I had never had a conversation about how people would or would not view me as a parent. I had never dreamed that someone might not see me as a parent. My whole world just came crashing down. I am usually quite good on my feet and would have a comment or a response to constructively deal with the situation but I couldn't even get my words out. Honestly AJ, I just folded. I just kept saying 'I am her mum' but my words were getting caught. In that moment, I was crushed, and it felt like my world had come tumbling down. I just had never prepared myself for anyone to dismiss me as her mother. Oh gosh sorry, it's got me all emotional now. Sorry.

AJ: Oh darling, please don't apologize, I am sorry that I've made you re-live that...

Laura: No, it's important, I am just hormonal and pregnant [laughing].

AJ: If you need to stop or move on just let me know and we can carry on when you are ready.

Laura: No, it's okay, I want people to know what happened. It's important for people to be aware of how others may address or even dismiss them, so they know how to handle it. Being a non-biological parent can be a difficult role for many and I want to highlight the stigma attached to it by openly sharing how difficult it is, without the feeling of guilt or shame.

AJ: Okay, so you were still in hospital when this happened?

Laura: Yes, and the nurse just sort of ushered me out, trying to be kind and holding on to me, you know. But as I looked back, she was mishandling the baby. I have seen how doctors do those checks. I saw them with our second child. I know how they are done. She was really being rough. I asked her to stop, and she just ignored me. I got some strength from somewhere to say it louder, 'You are going to hurt her; you need to stop.' She was holding her up and dropping her, aggressively. I just grabbed the baby, and the nurse took me out. I was crying. The nurse was apologetic, and I just couldn't understand why she would have treated the baby like that. The nurse apologized and said that is her way, she is always like that. She said she isn't very nice to most people, not just you. I said that isn't an excuse. The nurse said you can put in a complaint to the Patient and Advice Liaison Service (PALS), so obviously even the nurse thought she was treating me and the baby badly, you know?

AJ: Yeah, it sounds horrific. I know they must do that startle reflex test and it can look a bit concerning but it doesn't sound like that was all that was happening.

Laura: No not at all. I have seen that check done on many babies and

I have never seen anyone do it as aggressively or forcefully as this doctor did to her.

When I got back to my wife on the ward, she obviously had no idea what had happened and was trying to comfort me, and she was the one who had given birth the day before.

That experience really tainted the first 18 months of our daughter's life. I felt that I had to validate my connection with her the whole time, even at the supermarket when little old ladies would coo over her and ask who's her mum to us both standing there. When people in the street would stop – you know what it is like when you have a little baby, everyone wants to talk to them and see them – I must have looked like I had lost the plot to some people who would only talk to Stacey and say, 'You must be so proud, she's so cute.' I would interject with 'I am her mum too!' and I honestly look back and think I must have looked neurotic. I felt that since the day after she was born, everyone would be questioning my validity as a mother.

It took me a long time to get over that. I hadn't considered before that day that I wasn't her mum. I wasn't her parent. So, when the doctor questioned it, it really threw me.

AJ: Yeah, from the day after she was born.

Laura: Yes, then in contrast when our son was born, the doctor who came in to do those checks with him just asked us how we were doing, who we were, and said, 'How wonderful, I am so happy for you both.' I was a bit worried he might be rough with him too, given our previous experience. I thought I am going to watch this to see if it was me being a fragile new first-time mum last time, but he was so gentle and so kind.

AJ: What a comparison between two babies and two healthcare professionals, huh?

Laura: No, it wasn't the same at all. There was no care, she was so aggressive, whereas he was attentive, professional and empathetic. He really took the time to listen and learn more about our journey.

Experiences like that can really tarnish and change your relationship with each other and the baby. I became quite withdrawn. I wouldn't let people hold the baby, even when family came over I would be holding her most of the time. I really don't know how Stacey dealt with it at the time, to be honest. Now I look back at how she was with our son (who Laura carried and birthed), she wasn't like that, so I really think it must have been because from the start I felt invalidated as a mum.

We've had some great experiences over the years, but we have also encountered people who are horrible and homophobic, and it is a shame that it was our first experience that was tarnished because there are some amazing people out there who have cared for us so well.

Even during this pregnancy now, I have had to explain to people what a frozen IVF transfer is and it's a waste of their time and my time. I felt so bad for one midwife because I could see how uncomfortable it was making her that she had to keep apologizing and asking what this meant, what does this procedure entail, what is this medication for. I felt sorry for her and it was awkward at times, although I did tell her what work I do and that I don't mind answering any questions she has, but you could see how uncomfortable she was because she didn't know. She said 'I should know this' so many times. It isn't her fault.

AJ: It's not. It's not a part of the education that they get, so it isn't her fault. I have so many healthcare professionals who come to me off their own backs to do the workshop or ask questions and I do feel bad, because it should be a mandated part of their training.

Laura: Yes, it's not something that would cost billions of pounds to change either. In a lot of examples, it's just a case of having an awareness and thinking before you speak. It was harder this time, because we had IUI with our first two children, but then we had three rounds of IUI and they all failed, so we had a frozen IVF transfer for this pregnancy.

AJ: During a pandemic as well.

Laura: Yes, not the easiest route, was it? Because of my diminished ovarian reserve, we had to. We didn't know how much more time we had to try.

AJ: Your story is a really great example. It's horrific, don't get me wrong, but I think it perfectly captures so many of the struggles that LGBT+ parents have. We have to get in through the door, so our NHS trust has to agree to give funding, or we access sperm clinics and get all those aspects sorted. We try and it might fail, so we deal with that, and then finally it works and we're pregnant and then we still have to navigate the services of blatant everyday homophobia and the restrictions within the institution as well. It's not just the institution, it's the individuals within it as well.

Even when we have our babies, we are then dealing with homophobia or being erased with forms for schools, or at the doctor's office, wherever it might be. It's not as if when we have the baby, finally, homophobia, transphobia or biphobia stops.

Laura: It is this continual questioning, continually having to come out every time we take our child for a doctor's appointment. Then if it's a doctor who has no idea how we created our family I am met with all this questioning about how we conceived and if we know who the 'dad' is before they will look at my child who is poorly! As our children are getting older, it's worrying for them because they might grow up thinking it's normal for healthcare professionals to question their parents on everything about their conception, birth and family dynamics just to get an ear infection checked.

AJ: Exhausting!

Laura: It is. This isn't every time, but when we see a locum or a different doctor from our usual one there are always questions. It could all be avoided by them asking, 'Who is here today?' This open questioning could save so much back-pedalling when we have to explain who we are, and I feel that I am justifying myself each time. In some situations, it leaves the healthcare professional embarrassed at having to ask such intrusive questions.

AJ: Sometimes, healthcare professionals might have to ask these questions though, and I get that. It might be to rule out a genetic condition, or it might affect the measurements that a sonographer has taken to know the method of conception. I think most LGBT+ parents understand that. But it is *how* it is asked.

Laura: Yes, I agree, but even then, even if they ask perfectly and we are happy and feel loved and cared for and safe answering those questions, the healthcare professionals don't have the training to know what I am saying in some regards. They aren't educated in what a frozen transfer is, or what IUI is and how it is different from IVF. So, we end up having to explain it all anyway. It's a great thing to have a healthcare professional who is asking open questions, not making assumptions and really doing a great job on that side of things. However, it still leaves us having to explain ourselves one way or another.

AJ: That is true, good point.

Laura: They deserve that support. They are the ones that are working for the NHS and now really putting their lives on the line. They deserve to be given this education and training so they can care for us properly. That is what they want to do, in most of the cases.

Also, the back-office systems could be there for our children as well. There could be something on the files for children of LGBT+ families that explains how they were conceived, who is the biological/non-biological parent, what the donor's medical history is, if required, so that doctors don't have to ask them every time. There is no data collection on our community at present at all.

They then might not even have to ask who is here with you today because the information would be on the screen and that would cut down on the time taken in appointments for us to explain, and that would save the NHS money and time.

AJ: The data capture is just a whole other mess.

Laura: We ask at so many meetings why our data isn't being captured; it is something we are working towards changing. We see it that so many people are having caesarean births who might not have wanted them with fertility treatment, but because they aren't capturing that data, we can't say look X per cent of families using IVF had caesareans, why is that? We need to investigate that. Without data on our community and our needs, how can we be fully supported and given the personalized care each individual needs?

AJ: I had an interesting conversation with Dr Mari Greenfield about this, and I hope it will change soon and capturing gender and sexuality will happen so that healthcare professionals and families can be better informed.

Laura: When they collect the census data, it will be helpful but won't cover healthcare. The data isn't there, and until it is, we can't do much more.

AJ: Can we circle back to sperm donation?

Laura: Sure!

AJ: What is it that you want healthcare professionals to know about sperm donation?

Laura: We went to America for our sperm because you get more information and they have a greater choice of ethnicities, so we found it better to look in America.

We got a baby photo, an adult photo, his medical history, his family history, an essay of why he wanted to do it; everything, right down to the waves in his hair really! There was a lot more detail than you get through clinics in the UK.

There are a lot of assumptions that we don't have any information from our donor. We have to say sometimes we have medical history available if it's needed because the assumption is that we know nothing about him. It would be helpful for healthcare professionals to know the differences in the information that you are given when you use a sperm bank from a different country. If they had asked something like 'Can I ask if you used a sperm bank and, if so, was that in the UK?' then immediately, when we said, no it was in America, they would know that we most likely had a lot more information than if we said it was in the UK, they would again immediately know that we have limited information. Some people may use a known donor or their friend and might have that information. I think it would be helpful to have a general idea of what information people may or may not have.

AJ: Yeah, I agree, that could save time and some delicate conversations.

Laura: The thing is, I really don't mind chatting and answering questions. I have said to midwives before, 'I have loads of information about him. I even have pictures!' They get excited and want to have a look and that's fine. With what I do, I feel it's important that I am open and answer questions. However, that isn't going to be everyone's experience and not everyone will want to share all of this, due to being shy, private or having suffered trauma, so that is totally valid too.

Those midwives are usually then even happier for us because they have had an insight into our journey. They have seen what we have gone through and understand what an incredible experience we've been through and what a miracle it is that our babies are here.

AJ: It is incredible. It is beautiful. It should be celebrated and not something to shy away from through fear of getting it wrong. With just a bit of common sense and empathy it can be achieved because it is already happening!

Laura: Absolutely, absolutely.

*

Laura and her partner Stacey's third child was born in June 2021. They continue to be a powerhouse in the LGBT+ birth world. Laura is an incredible advocate for the LGBT+ community and a powerful ally to the trans and non-binary community.

CHAPTER 9

Conclusion

I have thought long and hard how I want this book to end. What is the takeaway message? What is the final word? Well sorry folks, there isn't one.

Most people I have spoken to have said they simply want acknowledgement that we exist. That it is possible a pregnant man will need you. It's possible there is no dad or mum.

As the world evolves and we continue to learn more about ourselves, and the world around us, this will one day be outdated. How could we have thought that there was only binary and non-binary – pfft, weirdos.

That's the game, that's how it is played, and you can't be upset by progress and growth.

There are many more battles on the horizon for all who birth their babies: the women, the people, the men. Gaining recognition for non-binary people and their gender or lack thereof is a big one that I can see coming to the forefront soon. With the advancements of science, trans women and indeed cis women who are otherwise unable to may be able to carry babies. With changes to the laws surrounding the GRC and self-identification, I hope most of what I've written will be wrong in a few years.

Further Reading and Resources

Podcast
NB – BBC Sounds

Films
Seahorse: The Dad Who Gave Birth
A Deal with the Universe

Books
Where's the Mother? – Trevor MacDonald
Pride and Joy: A Guide for Gay Bisexual and Trans Parents – Sarah and Rachel Hagger-Holt
Trans Like Me – CN Lester
Pregnant Butch – A.K. Summers

About the Author

AJ Silver is a birth and postnatal doula, who trained with Red Tent Doulas, Abuela Doulas and Badass Doulas. They are also a breastfeeding counsellor, as well as a qualified babywearing consultant with the School of Babywearing.

Their work within LGBT+ competency training in the UK has seen them running workshops, lecturing and speaking with universities, NHS trusts, groups and collectives of other birth workers.

If you are interested in attending a workshop, go to their website, The Queer Birth Club.

They live in Essex with their spouse of 12 years, two children and a springer spaniel called Princess Leia.

Coming out at the age of 15 as bisexual, they have long been an active and proud member of the LGBT+ community. During their pregnancy and birth, they began to question their gender identity, in part but not solely because of the overt genderfication of pregnancy, birth and early parenting.

They have featured on many podcasts and interviews and had their works published by AIMS (Association for the Improvement of Maternity Services).

For more information on the author please go to www.birthkeeperdoula.co.uk and https://queerbirthclub.co.uk.

Email: hello@queerbirthclub.co.uk

Facebook: www.facebook.com/thequeerbirthclub

Instagram: www.instagram.com/thequeerbirthclub

Abuela Doulas: https://abueladoulas.com
Badass Doulas: www.badassbirth.co.uk

Index